This book is dedicated to all the women who have in the past, do in the present, or will in the future, suffer the pain and consequences of pelvic inflammatory disease.

Preface

Pelvic Inflammatory Disease (PID) continues to be a major public health concern, with over one million cases diagnosed annually in the United States, at a cost of over $4 billion. In addition, PID is the most frequent cause of hospitalization among reproductive age women. The disease is usually associated with sexually transmitted organisms and organisms that constitute the flora of the vagina, specifically anaerobic and facultative organisms. In young women, approximately two thirds of PID is caused by, or associated with, chlamydia and/or gonorrhoeae. Recent evidence has demonstrated that bacterial vaginosis also plays an important role in the pathogenesis of PID.

The morbidity associated with acute PID, however, does not reside solely with the acute illness. Long-term consequences even after a single episode of PID result from fallopian tube damage and include tubal-factor infertility, ectopic pregnancy, and chronic pelvic pain. Although Swedish studies have demonstrated infertility in 16% of PID patients, studies from Canada and the United States reported a higher rate of infertility following acute PID. Women are also at a seven- to tenfold increased risk for ectopic pregnancy following PID.

Of increasing concern is the growing body of data indicating that a substantial proportion of cases of PID are unrecognized and, therefore, untreated. The term "unrecognized PID" is suggested for those upper genital tract infections that are asymptomatic or are not associated with the classic signs and symptoms suggestive of acute PID. The diagnosis of unrecognized PID is established in women with inflammation of the upper genital tract (endometrium and/or fallopian tubes) in the absence of abdominal pain. Most importantly, unrecognized PID causes similar long-term sequelae to acute symptomatic PID, specifically ectopic pregnancy formation and tubal factor infertility. Risk factors for and clinical predictors of unrecognized PID have yet to be elucidated, making this a fertile area for future research efforts. Identification of risk factors/markers for the development of PID have been the focus of increasing attention. Age is an important risk factor for PID and is inversely related to PID rates. Of particular concern are adolescent females who are at significant risk of developing acute salpingitis.

Contraception practices significantly affect the risk for PID. Women using oral contraceptive agents or barrier methods, such as condoms and diaphragms, appear to have protection from upper genital tract infection. On the other hand, use of the intrauterine contraceptive device (IUD) and lack of contraception increase the risk of PID. In addition, vaginal douching has been implicated in the development of PID along with sex during menses.

Establishing factors to predict upper genital tract infection would have substantial implications for the health of reproductive-aged women. Moreover, reliable predictors of unrecognized PID may alert the clinician to be more aggressive in treatment and follow-up of these patients. This may result in timely treatment of PID, which would be an important factor in reducing the consequences of PID. Among women in the United States today, PID remains among the most significant and consequential repercussion of the STD epidemic. This book is aimed at providing a comprehensive resource book on PID by leading authors and researchers in the field.

Daniel V. Landers
Richard L. Sweet

Contents

Preface vii

Contributors xi

1 Epidemiology of Pelvic Inflammatory Disease 1
   David A. Eschenbach

2 Risk Factors for Pelvic Inflammatory Disease and
   Associated Sequelae 21
   Nancy S. Padian and A. Eugene Washington

3 Microbial Etiology of Pelvic Inflammatory Disease 30
   Richard L. Sweet

4 Diagnosis of Pelvic Inflammatory Disease 60
   Pål Wølner-Hanssen

5 Treatment of Acute Pelvic Inflammatory Disease 76
   Richard L. Sweet

6 Tubo-Ovarian Abscess Complicating Pelvic
   Inflammatory Disease 94
   Daniel V. Landers

7 Pelvic Inflammatory Disease in Pregnancy 107
   Joseph G. Pastorek II

8 Pelvic Inflammatory Disease in the Adolescent Female 116
   Vivien Igra, Jonathan Ellen, and Mary-Ann Shafer

9 Pelvic Inflammatory Disease and HIV-1 Infection 139
   Abner P. Korn and Daniel V. Landers

10   Prevention of Pelvic Inflammatory Disease 146
      Julius Schachter

11   Long-term Sequelae of Pelvic Inflammatory Disease:
      Tubal Factor Infertility, Ectopic Pregnancy,
      and Chronic Pelvic Pain 152
      Joan M. Chow and Julius Schachter

12   Histopathology of Genital Tract Infection with *C. trachomatis*
      and *N. gonorrhoeae* 170
      Nancy Kiviat

13   Behavioral Aspects of Pelvic Inflammatory Disease 181
      Stuart N. Seidman and Sevgi Okten Aral

Index   205

Contributors

Sevgi Okten Aral, Ph.D.
Associate Director for Science, Division of STD Prevention, Centers for Disease Control, Atlanta, GA 30333, USA

Joan M. Chow, Dr. P.H.
Assistant Research Epidemiologist, Department of Laboratory Medicine, San Francisco General Hospital, San Francisco, CA 94110, USA

Jonathan Ellen, M.D.
Division of Adolescent Medicine, University of California at San Francisco, San Francisco, CA 94143, USA

David A. Eschenbach, M.D.
Professor and Chief, Division of Gynecology, Department of Obstetrics and Gynecology, University of Washington, Seattle, WA 98195, USA

Vivien Igra, M.D.
Division of Adolescent Medicine, University of California at San Francisco, San Francisco, CA 94143, USA

Nancy Kiviat, M.D.
Professor of Pathology and Director, Cytopathology Laboratory, University of Washington, Seattle, WA 98195, USA

Abner P. Korn, M.D.
Associate Clinical Professor, University of California at San Francisco, and Director, Division of Gynecology, San Francisco General Hospital, San Francisco, CA 94110, USA

Daniel V. Landers, M.D.
Associate Professor and Director, Division of Reproductive Infectious Diseases and Immunology, Department of Obstetrics, Gynecology, and Reproductive Sciences, University of Pittsburgh School of Medicine, Magee-Women's Hospital, Pittsburgh, PA 15213-3180, USA

Nancy S. Padian, Ph.D.
Associate Professor and Assistant Chief of Research, Department of Obstetrics Gynecology, and Reproductive Sciences, University of California at San Francisco, San Francisco, CA 94143, USA

Joseph G. Pastorek II, M.D.
Professor and Chief, Section of Infectious Diseases, Department of Obstetrics-Gynecology, Louisiana State University School of Medicine, New Orleans, LA 70112, USA

Julius Schachter, Ph.D.
Professor and Director, Chlamydia Laboratories, Department of Laboratory Medicine, University of California at San Francisco, and San Francisco General Hospital, San Francisco, CA 94110, USA

Stuart N. Seidman, M.D.
341 West 87 Street, New York, NY 10024, USA

Mary-Ann Shafer, M.D.
Professor and Associate Director, Division of Adolescent Medicine, University of California at San Francisco, San Francisco, CA 94143, USA

Richard L. Sweet, M.D.
Professor and Chairman, Department of Obstetrics, Gynecology, and Reproductive Sciences, University of Pittsburgh School of Medicine, Magee-Women's Hospital, Pittsburgh, PA 15213-3180, USA

A. Eugene Washington, M.D., M.Sc.
Professor and Chairman, Department of Obstetrics, Gynecology, and Reproductive Sciences, University of California at San Francisco, San Francisco, CA 94143, USA

Pål Wølner-Hanssen, M.D.
Associate Professor, Department of Obstetrics and Gynecology, University of Lund, University Hospital, S-221 85 Lund, Sweden

1
Epidemiology of Pelvic Inflammatory Disease

DAVID A. ESCHENBACH

Pelvic inflammatory disease (PID) is the most common serious infection of women. Pelvic inflammatory disease is a cause of about 30% of infertility, 50% of ectopic pregnancies, and it is one of the most common causes of potentially preventable chronic pelvic pain. Pelvic inflammatory disease is not a reportable disease in the United States and precise figures on its prevalence are not available. Based upon a variety of sources, it is estimated that 10% to 15% of reproductive age women have had one episode of PID.[1] An estimated 750,000 new cases occur annually.[2] The rate of PID is highly dependent on age. Among teenagers, an annual 1.5% incidence occurred in Lund, Sweden during the 1970s.[3] In the United States, black women have nearly twice the rate of PID as white women.[1] Between 1982 and 1988, a drop occurred in the cumulative rate of PID in all demographic groups except for white teenagers.[1] There was also an encouraging drop in hospitalization for multiple episodes of PID during this span.

The majority of PID is related to the recovery of two sexually transmitted bacteria, *Neisseria gonorrhoeae* and *Chlamydia trachomatis*. The number of infections that are estimated to occur from *N. gonorrhoeae* has decreased since 1985.[4] This drop in rates of gonorrhoeae may in part account for the drop in rates of PID seen during this period. Less is known about the trend of *C. trachomatis* infection in the U.S. However, marked decreases in the rate of PID have followed widespread chlamydia screening programs in Sweden and parts of the U.S. when rates of chlamydia infection fall. Factors associated with the acquisition of these two bacteria are in turn associated with PID. Other factors, contraceptive use, douching practices, cigarette smoking, and recurrent infection have additional impact upon the development of PID independent of these bacteria.

Thus, epidemiology of PID is complex. Pelvic inflammatory disease can be considered a complication of cervical infection. Factors that influence cervical infection directly affect PID. To date, the epidemiology of PID has not been examined separately from that of cervical infection. It will be incumbent upon investigation to begin to separate factors that effect cervical infection and PID in future studies.

Cervical infection is often, but not always, caused by sexually transmitted microorganisms. The epidemiology of infection with sexually transmitted microorganisms is complex itself. True causal factors for the acquisition of a sexually transmitted disease (STD) are largely dependent upon the chance of encountering an infected partner, or the rate of exposure. Other causal factors influence the rate of acquisition once exposed, of developing disease once infected, and of progression of disease into advanced stages once disease occurs.[5] Some causal factors potentially effect more than one of these levels, although solid data is frequently absent and many of the hypothesis presented lack solid evidence of the exact level they influence. Quantitation of the importance of one factor relative to another has usually not been documented. To further complicate this issue, another large group of factors appear to represent only surrogates of causal factors and as such represent confounding factors or risk markers rather than true causal factors. Low socioeconomic status (SES) is an example of a confounding factor rather than a causal factor for cervical infection and PID. Low SES women with PID may appear to have increased exposure, acquisition, development, or progression of the infection. However, low SES per se is not causally related to any of these levels. Rather, low SES represents a surrogate for individuals whose sexual behavior or health-care behavior increase the rate of PID by increasing the causal factors of encountering infection, developing disease once exposed, or having progression of disease. For some factors, it is not clear whether the factor represents a causal or a confounding factor (or both).[5]

Ultimately, these causal factors have to influence the microorganisms that cause infection or the defense mechanisms of that infection that affect disease. Again, we are at a disadvantage, because the pathogenesis of cervical infection and of PID is incompletely understood. Despite the uncertainties over whether certain factors are causal factors or confounding factors and over the pathogenesis, it is helpful in the understanding of PID to consider factors in the pathogenesis of first cervical infection and then PID.

Socioeconomic Status, Marital Status, Race, and Drug Use

Individuals in a low SES group, single and divorced women, blacks and other minorities in the United States, and individuals who abuse drugs and alcohol have had higher rates of *N. gonorrhoeae* and PID.[6-8] These demographic and behavioral factors undoubtedly represent surrogates for sexual behavior. These confounding factors identify groups at high risk of acquiring cervical infection, but none of these factors independently explain why patients would have increased rates of infection. SES, marital status, race, and drug use per se do not cause the high infection rates in these groups. These factors are in turn associated with the chance of exposure to sexually transmitted bacteria and other bacteria that cause PID.

Age

The highest rate of PID is found among sexually active women between the ages of 15 and 25.[9-11] PID rates are low for patients over the age of 35. Teenagers, in particular, have had high rates of PID.[1]

Several biological explanations exist to explain why age could be a causal factor for PID. Increased estrogen levels following menarche causes an expansion in the area of columnar epithelium on the cervical portio. Young patients typically have large areas of cervical ectopy, which gradually regress as squamous epithelium and eventually overgrows the columnar epithelium.[12] Young women have larger areas of ectopy than older women. Patients with a large area of cervical ectopy have a greater area for *N. gonorrhoeae* and *C. trachomatis* to attach. Patients using oral contraceptives have a larger zone of ectopy and a higher rate of *C. trachomatis* than those using other contraception. Thus, large areas of cervical ectopy could increase the rate of cervical acquisition of bacteria, and, in turn, PID. Ectopy appears to be a stronger predictor than oral contraceptive use of *C. trachomatis* infection[13] and high *C. trachomatis* inclusion counts.[14] Young patients would also be expected to have fewer ovulatory menstrual cycles than patients in their twenties. The presence of estrogen without the presence of progesterone produces abundant cervical mucus that potentially allows sperm, and perhaps bacteria, to more readily move through cervical mucus than in the presence of progesterone, which causes a complex matrix of cervical mucus.[15] Further, young patients would be expected to be less likely to have serum and local antibody to cervical pathogens. Specific antibodies may offer protection against the attachment of bacteria or protection against infection of the tubes among those with cervical infection.[16]

However, young sexually active patients also have a higher number of sexual partners than older patients.[17] Teenagers have had particularly high rates of *N. gonorrhoeae* and *C. trachomatis*. Thus, age could represent a confounding factor related to sexual activity leading to a higher rate of cervical infection because of exposure to a greater number of sexual partners. In this scenario, age does not account for a direct effect upon cervical or tubal infection. Teenagers remained with a high rate of PID after controlling for sexual activity in one study,[18] but cervical *N. gonorrhoeae* and *C. trachomatis* infection were not controlled in this small sample. We found no relationship between age and the rate of PID when patients with gonococcal PID were compared to patients with asymptomatic gonorrhea.[19] Similarly, age was not related to PID when patients with chlamydial PID were compared to patients with asymptomatic chlamydia. The presence of these two cervical pathogens appears to be more important than age in the development of PID. These two cervical pathogens appear to be more important than the zone of cervical ectopy, anovulatory estrogen dominant cycles, and antibody in producing PID.

Sexual Behavior

Sexual behavior has been measured by the number of current and lifetime sexual partners, age of first intercourse, frequency of intercourse, selection and duration of partners, and types of sexual practice. The number of recent sexual partners has been associated with cervical *N. gonorrhoeae*[20] and *C. trachomatis* infection.[21,22] Multiple, particularly new sexual partners would be expected to increase acquisition of these two sexually transmitted bacteria. Patients with new sexual partners and recent onset of lower genital tract symptoms may be particularly likely to attend STD clinics and be detected by these studies. The study of the relationship between STDs and sexual behavior is not straightforward because usually only one of the sexual behaviors parameters is studied. In addition, data usually are not included on the sexual activity of the male sexual partner.

Multiple recent sexual partners has been associated with PID.[6,8,23] In fact, multiple sexual partners has a relatively high risk ratio for presence of PID.[6,23] A new sexual partner in the prior month was also related to PID.[24] Multiple recent partners or a new partner could increase the exposure to infectious agents and acquisition of cervical infection. While multiple partners is a risk factor for acquisition of cervical infection, it may not be a factor in causing PID independent of cervical infection. Sexual behavior among patients with and without PID has not been controlled for the two cervical pathogens (*N. gonorrhoeae* and *C. trachomatis*) associated with cervical infection and PID.

The frequency of intercourse has been associated with PID in some,[6,8,24,25] but not all studies.[23] Increased frequency of intercourse could increase cervical exposure to a pathogen, upset vaginal homeostasis allowing overgrowth of virulent vaginal bacteria, increase the introduction of perineal pathogens into the vaginal canal, or increase patient exposure to bacteria attached to sperm.[26,27] Further study is required to determine if the frequency of intercourse is a risk factor for PID independent of the presence of cervical gonorrhea and chlamydia.

Males with untreated *N. gonorrhoeae* and *C. trachomatis* represent reservoirs for initial and recurrent cervical infections. Only about 20% of male sexual contacts of women with PID sought therapy for urethritis prior to the development of PID in their female partner.[28,29] About 60% of male contacts of women with PID and gonorrhea, including 80% of symptomatic men and 40% of asymptomatic men, had *N. gonorrhoeae* isolated from the urethra.[29] This finding suggests that patients with PID have recently acquired gonorrhea and, further, suggests that most of the male contacts infected with gonorrhea are either asymptomatic or have minimal symptoms that fail to reliably bring them to treatment. Of male partners of women with PID in whom *N. gonorrhoeae* was not isolated, 10% has *N. gonorrhoeae* and 10% had nongonococcal urethritis,[29] an infection where about half of the men have *C. trachomatis*. Infected male sexual partners of women with PID are important in the acquisition of the original pathogen and are important in explaining the high recurrence of infection noted in some studies. Identification and treatment of male sexual partners of women with PID is necessary to reduce recurrent infection.

Health-Care Behavior

Health-care behavior has not received much attention as it relates to PID. Complex models of health behavior exist and these models become even more complex when involving STDs.[30] Briefly, features of health-care behavior include a perception of illness, knowledge of the disease, accessibility to care, and a medical evaluation on which is superimposed social and economic factors. Prompt recognition and presentation for diagnosis and treatment of cervical infection is important to reduce the development of PID. Prompt attention would be expected also to reduce the chance that cervical infection progresses to the serious stage of PID.

Most investigators who study women in low SES groups with PID are impressed that their perception of the illness and the potential consequences of sequellae is often limited. Patients in low SES groups may not be aware of the importance of symptoms in the recognition of disease and may not realize that delays may cause not only tubal infection, but tubal infection leads to tubal infertility. Accessibility to medical care is diminished by high costs and a mistrust of the medical system. Many women are the head of households today. A woman responsible for shelter, clothing, and food for the family may perceive her health to be of secondary importance to these responsibilities and additionally, may have little time or energy to provide basic health care for herself. A perception that health is secondary to other duties acts to delay diagnosis and treatment. Such a perception further impacts antibiotic compliance, return check-ups, and notification and treatment of partners—issues important in the development of recurrent infection.

On the other hand, health-care behavior is probably less important for patients who develop fallopian tube infection with minimal or no symptoms. It is now apparent that the majority of patients with PID have symptoms so common or so mild that they do not seek therapy for PID.[31] Although the rate of PID is highest in low SES groups, a large proportion of PID still occurs in the greater number of patients in other economic groups. Studies of tubal infertility among patients in middle or high SES groups has made it apparent that most PID occurs with few or minimal symptoms. About two-thirds of patients with tubal infertility in multiple reports have not received treatment for PID.[31] In these reports, tubal fertility was recorded among patients with the financial backing or the medical sophistication to undergo tests that identify tubal infertility in these reports. Many patients with tubal infertility, particularly those with limited funds and/or knowledge of health care, have not been studied. It is possible that health-care behavior is less of an issue in the development of PID among patients in whom PID occurs relatively asymptomatically. It is important to study whether the same amount of asymptomatic PID occurs in the low SES group. If less asymptomatic PID occurred in the low SES group (because of higher *N. gonorrhoeae* rates, for example) health-care behavior attitudes become relatively more important for that group. Alternatively, if the same high rate of asymptomatic PID occurs in the low SES group, as was reported in other SES groups, programs that increase health-care awareness would have significantly less impact on PID and prevention of PID would focus on screening for asymptomatic cervical infection, for example. Further study is required to clarify this important issue.

Cigarette Smoking

Cigarette smoking has been associated with cervical gonorrhea and other STDs. Patients who continue to smoke after knowing the health risks of smoking may be risk-takers who acquire more STDs and who have poor health-care seeking behavior. These patients would be expected to take more risks with sex leading to a greater number of partners, to have less knowledge of whether their sexual partners are symptomatic with infection or have other partners, to less often use barrier contraception that would protect against infection, and to have a low chance of seeking care for symptoms.

If cigarette smoking is related to acquisition of STDs, it then is not surprising to find that cigarette smoking has recently been associated with PID.[32] Current and previous smoking was found twice as common in patients with PID than controls after adjusting for 8 variables associated with PID in that population.[32] Unfortunately, presence of cervical *N. gonorrhoeae* and *C. trachomatis* were not controlled in the report. There was no dose–response relationship observed between smoking and PID. Thus, it is not known if cigarette smoking is a causal factor in the development of PID independent of the link between smoking and cervical infection. The relative risk of PID among former smokers was slightly higher than the relative risk of PID among current smokers,[32] raising the possibility that smoking and PID were related through some indirect association such as cervical infection.

Smoking has been related to tubal infertility with a relative risk of 2 to 3,[33,34] but not to other reasons for infertility.[34] The relative risk of tubal infertility was increased in smoking over nonsmoking patients in analyses stratified for those who ever used an intrauterine device (IUD) or oral contraceptives, suggesting that smoking was independent of contraception in its relationship with tubal infertility.[33] Smoking exerted a dose–response effect (pack–years and age smoking began) on infertility caused by cervical factor and tubal disease.[33] Smoking also has been related to ectopic pregnancy, but a dose–response effect was not found for ectopic pregnancy.[35] Tubal infertility and ectopic pregnancy are sequellae of PID and it is tempting to conclude that cigarette smoking is causally related to PID.

Metabolites from smoking are present in the cervical mucus of smokers.[36] These metabolites could be toxic to sperm causing cervical factor infertility and they could also depress local immunity increasing the chance of infection spreading beyond the cervix. Tubal motility is reduced by smoking,[37] which could limit clearing of bacteria from the tubes. Cigarette smoking decreases cervical mucus killer cell activity[38] and the general immune response.[39] Smoking increases the risk of human immunodeficiency virus type 1 infection in women after controlling for sexual, marital, and religious factors.[40] These data suggest smoking may have an effect upon the ability of the immune system to limit attachment, invasion, or multiplication of microorganisms. On the other hand, evidence that smoking has an antiestrogen effect is quite strong.[41] Pelvic inflammatory disease is unusually among premenarchal and postmenopausal women, suggesting some effect of normal reproductive age ovarian function on PID. Anovulatory cycles have high estrogen levels and high estrogen levels may increase the possibility of PID. Estradiol is suspected of prolonging and increasing the ascent of chlamydial genital infection in guinea pigs.[42,43] Further research is required because of the large number of women who smoke cigarettes combined with a twofold increased risk of PID among smokers means that smoking is potentially an important population attributable risk for PID. Factors with a high population attributable risk means that a significant proportion of PID would be attributed to smoking.

Douching

Vaginal douching appears to be a common practice. About one-third of women over 18 douched within 1 week of a 1984 survey.[44] Limited data suggested douching may prevent vaginal infection.[45] Douching is probably ineffective in treating vaginal infection.

Vaginal douching has recently been associated with PID.[46,47] Women with PID were 1.7 times more likely to have douched in the previous 2 months than controls without PID in a multifactorial analysis in which demographic factors and cervical infection was controlled.[47] Cervical infection with N.

gonorrhoeae or *C. trachomatis* did not seem to influence the relationship between douching and PID. Douching 3 or more times per month was 3 to 4 times more common in the PID than the control group in an adjusted analysis, suggesting a dose–response.[47] The association between douching and PID was strongest for those with fewer lifetime sexual partners, indicating that douching may be factor for PID among women at low risk to develop PID. In fact, douching was related to PID among white, but not among black women, raising the possibility that douching was an independent risk factor among patients at lower risk for PID. Commercial disposable units seemed to be particularly associated with PID.[47] Douching may alter the microbiological environment of the vagina by increasing virulent bacteria. Douching could also flush fluid or vaginal bacteria into the uterine and tubal spaces to increase the potential for the development of PID.

Douching has been related to ectopic pregnancy, a complication of PID. Weekly douching with a commercial preparation was 4 times more common among patients with an ectopic pregnancy than fertile women.[48] Further studies are required to establish if douching is a causal factor in PID. In the meantime, because douching has no proven medical benefit, it seems reasonable to recommend women not douche.

Menstruation

Patients with PID and *N. gonorrhoeae* tend to develop lower abdominal pain within the first part of the menstrual cycle, particularly the first week following the onset of menses.[49,50] The same relationship occurs for *C. trachomatis*. The onset of pain began within the first 7 days of menses in one-half of patients with *N. gonorrhoeae* and/or *C. trachomatis* and 15% of patients with neither bacteria.[50] The onset of pain began 14 or more days after menses for one-half of those with neither bacteria. These findings suggest menses is a factor for either the dissemination or multiplication of gonorrhea and chlamydia in the endometrium and/or fallopian tubes. Cervical mucus is lost during menses. Cervical mucus acts as a mechanical barrier,[15] particularly among patients who ovulate and produce progesterone. Progesterone causes a dense matrix of the cervical mucus, which limits sperm and probably bacterial entry into the uterine cavity. The cervical mucus also contains immunoglobulins, which perhaps presents an immunologic barrier to bacteria in the lower genital tract.

Blood during menses provides a good substrate for bacterial growth. Virulent gonococci become more common during menses than other phases of the menstrual cycle.[51] These findings are also consistent with the observation that little PID develops among women using intramuscular progesterone for contraception (L. Weström, personal communication). Patients with IUDs containing progesterone have had less PID than other

IUD users. Patients on progesterone would have increased cervical mucus density and less bleeding with menses. It is important to identify if progesterone reduces the rate of PID and if it does whether the mechanism is through an effect upon cervical mucus, reduced menstrual blood, or some other direct effect upon the microorganisms or cellular attachment.

Prior and Present Infection

Prior PID

A previous episode of PID is a risk for the development of subsequent PID. A patient with PID was 2.3 times more likely than a patient without PID to have a history of previous PID in a discriminate analysis of a population where multiple sexual partners, African-American ancestry, and IUD use were also related to PID.[23] About one-quarter of patients with a documented episode of PID develop a subsequent PID episode.[52]

Factors important in the development of subsequent PID could include repetitive infections from untreated male sexual partners, inadequate antibiotic therapy, or sexual behavior. It is further possible that tubal damage from one episode of PID leads to a certain rate of tubal infection from nonsexually transmitted microorganisms. There are no direct data on the possibility of whether bacteria commonly enter the uterus and fallopian tubes during menses. Female patients undergoing peritoneal dialysis because of kidney failure usually have blood from the endometrium noted in the abdomen during menses. Women with normal fallopian tubes would seldom develop infection from this phenomenon, while those with damaged tubes could be susceptible to tubal infection. Tubal epithelium previously damaged by infection is noted to have persistent chronic inflammation, reduction of cilia, and damage of surface epithelium[53]; these changes would be expected to increase susceptibility of the tube to infection, from even normal genital flora. Subsequent PID is important to prevent because tubal occlusion increases from 11% after one, to 23% after two, and 54% after three episodes of PID.[3]

An episode of *C. trachomatis* tubal infection following a prior episode of chlamydial PID may be particularly damaging to the fallopian tube. The first experimental *C. trachomatis* tubal infection in primates produces a self-limited infection. A polymorphonuclear leukocytes inflammatory response occurs, but it spontaneously subsided in 2 to 5 weeks without gross tubal damage. However, after repetitive inoculation of *C. trachomatis* into the fallopian tube, there was the sudden production of a severe tissue reaction where the tubes became occluded and peritubal adhesions occurred. A mononuclear inflammatory response was present in the repetitive infections.[54] Similar tissue damage occurs following repetitive inoculation of *C. trachomatis* into the eye. It is the current hypothesis that repetitive inoculation of *C. trachomatis* leads to a hyperimmune response where an over-reaction of the immune response (delayed hypersensitivity) produces the tissue damage.

Prior Gonorrhea

A history of previous cervical gonococcal infection without apparent PID has been found more commonly among patients with PID than controls.[8] This association could be related to the high rate of subsequent gonococcal infection among those with gonorrhea. Some core populations have very high recidivism of gonorrhea.[55] Such individuals would be at high risk for PID because they again acquire. *N. gonorrhoeae*. Another explanation is that some women with cervical *N. gonorrhoeae* infection develop subclinical tubal infection. If some patients developed unrecognized tubal infection at the time of cervical gonorrhea infection, they would be at high risk to develop PID for the same reason (prior tubal damage) that patients who developed overt PID have a high rate of subsequent infection. In fact, histologic changes among infertile women with tubal occlusion are similar in those without and with a prior history of PID.[53]

A prior episode of gonococcal PID appears to protect against a subsequent episode of gonococcal PID if infection occurs with the same antigenic principal outer membrane protein (POMP).[16] However, about one-half of subsequent infections involved a different POMP strain than was isolated from the original PID episode. Approximately 50% of women infected with a different POMP gonococcal stain went on to develop PID. Additionally, prior episodes of cervical gonorrhea without salpingitis may not stimulate enough antibodies to protect against PID, or immunity may be inferred only for short times.

Prior Chlamydia

Repeated experimental cervical inoculations of *C. trachomatis* produced tubal edema in the majority and uterine erythema in all animals.[56] Peritubal adhesions were found in all four animals who received weekly inoculations of *C. trachomatis* for 5 weeks. Tubal inoculation following repetitive cervical inoculation resulted in prominent tubal adhesions while tubal inoculation without prior cervical inoculation resulted in only minor adhesion formation.[56] These experiments demonstrate that repetitive cervical inoculation may produce increasingly severe tubal damage, similar to the data presented above in which repetitive tubal inoculations produced an acceleration of tubal damage.

Women with gonorrhea have a high prevalence of chlamydia.[57] To test whether gonorrhea reactivates a latent chlamydial infection, episodes of recurrent chlamydial infection were studied for the presence of gonorrhea. Serotyping of isolates revealed the presence of the same chlamydial serovar isolate in the first and second infection significantly more often in patients with concomitant gonorrhea (47%) than in patients without gonorrhea (23%).[57] This data suggests that chlamydial infection may be reactivated by a new gonococcal infection. To date, data suggests that patients with PID have had higher than expected rates of prior asymptomatic cervical chlamydial infection.[24] These findings even raise the intriguing possibility that a new cervical gonococcal infection can reactivate a latent chlamydial tubal infection.

Contraception

Barrier Methods

Condom and diaphragm use often with a spermicidal agent protects against the acquisition of cervical gonococcal infection.[58–60] Barrier method contraceptive use also had a significant protection against PID ($RR = 0.6$).[61] Condoms, diaphragms, and spermicides all provided similar protection against PID. These data suggest that barrier and spermicidal methods reduce the rate of salpingitis by reducing exposure to bacteria causing PID.

Oral Contraceptives

The effect of oral contraceptives on PID is complex. Oral contraceptives are associated with an increased risk of cervical chlamydia (but not cervical gonorrhea), a decreased risk of PID, and no effect on tubal infertility.

Oral contraceptive users generally have been found to have a two- to threefold increased risk of cervical chlamydia compared to other contraceptive users.[62,63] As previously mentioned, oral contraceptive use is also associated with cervical ectopy. The relationship between oral contraceptive use, ectopy, and chlamydia is complex[62] and not well understood. Cervical ectopy may provide a greater area for attachment of the bacteria to columnar epithelium and thus, ectopy could be related to acquisition of chlamydia. However, a larger area of ectopy may also make identification of chlamydia more likely. In fact, higher inclusion counts were present in those with rather than without ectopy,[14] suggesting that it would be easier to identify C. trachomatis in patients with ectopy. Adjustment for ectopy cancelled the effect of the ectopy on chlamydial isolation in one study,[62] but not in another.[13] At present, it is unclear if oral contraceptive use increases the infection rate or only identification of chlamydia.

Oral contraceptives are associated with a 50% decrease in PID in most studies,[6,8,64] but this finding is sometimes absent. Among patients with a clinical diagnosis of PID, laparoscopic confirmation of acute salpingitis is less often present in oral contraceptive users than in nonoral contraceptive users.[65] In addition, oral contraceptive users who had salpingitis observed at laparoscopy were less likely to have severe tubal disease compared to users of IUDs or no contraception.[66] Recently, oral contraceptives seemed to protect against PID in a subgroup of patients with chlamydial infection alone ($OR = 0.2$), but not for patients with gonorrhea alone ($OR = 0.9$).[24] Patients with gonorrhea and chlamydia and those with neither microorganism seemed to have some protection against PID, but the protection from oral contraceptive use was not significant. Multivariate adjustment for potentially confounding demographic and behavioral factors did not change the association.[24] Others have reported a protective effect of oral contraceptive use for patients with gonococcal PID,[67,68] but the effect on chlamydial infection was not simultaneously examined in these studies. It has been suggested that the protective effect of oral contraceptives on PID is produced by changes in the cervical mucus, preventing bacterial ascent into the uterus or by an endometrial effect resulting in less menstrual bleeding or bacteria attachment. The protection against chlamydial but not gonococcal PID suggests oral contraceptive may cause a specific effect by reducing the susceptibility of upper genital tract mucosal cells to *C. trachomatis* or by down-regulating the delayed hypersensitivity immune response to chlamydia.

However, a word of caution is in order. As noted previously, oral contraceptive use may potentially increase the risk of chlamydial infections of the cervix. If oral contraceptives decrease the rate of chlamydial PID, there may be no net effect of oral contraception on chlamydial PID. In fact, tubal infertility is not influenced by prior oral contraceptive use,[34,69] suggesting the oral contraceptive does not exhibit a net protection against the sequellae of tubal disease.

Intrauterine Device

A causal link between the IUD and PID is based upon controlled studies in which IUD use was consistently more common in patients with PID than controls without PID,[70,71] together with clinical reports linking foreign bodies in general and the IUD in particular with infection.[72–74] As expected, tubal infertility is also related to IUD use.[34,69,75]

Case-control studies have consistently demonstrated a higher risk of PID for IUD users than users of other contraception or no contraception. The magnitude of this risk varies, but in most studies ranges from two- to fourfold. The magnitude of risk is less when the control group is noncontraceptive users than when the control group is all non-IUD users.[76] On the surface, noncontraceptive users appear to be a good control group because oral contraceptive and barrier users have a reduced rate of PID. However, individuals willing to risk using no contraception may be willing to take higher risks in areas not measured in these studies such as choice of partner, medical care for symptoms, and other risks related to PID and health care, such as smoking. Thus, individuals using no contraception may have increased rates of cervical gonorrhea and chlamydia or take health-care risks and be at increased risk for PID through this mechanism. The use of patients using no contraception as the control group underestimates the risk of PID in IUD users. The ideal control group does not exist for the examination of the role of contraception in PID, but perhaps the best control group is a composite of all other non-IUD using patients.

One large prospective study of 3162 IUD users found IUD users had a 3 to 3.5 increased rate of PID compared to non-IUD users.[77] Numerous other prospective studies of IUD use have been published,[78] but in most, control groups using other contraception have not been simultaneously followed, patient drop-out is considerable, and the studies nearly uniformly had no mechanism by which PID could be reliably identified or recorded. Thus, PID rates reported in most prospective studies of IUD use is so low that the reports are too unreliable to use for the study of PID.

There appears to be two general mechanisms of infection. One involves the transport of bacteria from the cervix and vagina into the uterine cavity during insertion.[79] The uterine cavity is usually sterile. Bacteria are isolated from the endometrium for the first 24 to 48 hours after insertion.[79] It was first reported that bacteria are usually not present 48 hours or more beyond insertion.[79] This mechanisms leads to the well agreed upon increase of PID for the first 4 to 6 months after insertion.[80]

The other mechanism is more complex. Following insertion, bacteria are grossly cleared from the uterine cavity. However, using more sensitive culture methods, it is now apparent that the presence of the IUD allows the wicking of bacteria along the tail and body.[72] As with other foreign bodies, bacteria attach to the surface of the IUD and cover themselves with a mucopolysaccharide.[81] The mechanical covering of bacteria prevents uterine defense mechanisms from eliminating bacteria off the surface of the IUD. In some individuals, virulent bacteria probably proliferate and disseminate from the IUD into the tubes to produce PID.

Intrauterine device users more commonly have higher than expected counts of anaerobic bacteria in the vagina,[82,83] including, for long-term IUD users, *Actinomyces*.[73] Intrauterine device users have bacteria isolated from the endometrium more commonly than non-IUD users.[84] Tailed IUDs are particularly associated with intrauterine bacteria.[72]

The IUD also apparently helps disseminate *N. gonorrhoeae* and *C. trachomatis*. Pelvic inflammatory disease rates are increased in IUD users with these two cervical infections over that expected. Intrauterine device users have the same rate of cervical *N. gonorrhoeae*[85,86] and *C. trachomatis*[83] as other contraceptive or no contraceptive users. However, IUD users with cervical gonorrhea or chlamydia have increased rates of PID. The increased rates of PID found are not related to overdiagnosis of PID in IUD users, because the clinical diagnosis of PID in IUD users is as accurate as in patients using no contraception.[66] Patients with gonorrhea have had a 3 to

6 times higher rate of PID than users of no contraception with gonorrhea.[8,85] The rate of IUD usage in patients with *C. trachomatis* and PID has been increased above expected. The proportion of patients with *C. trachomatis* is similar in IUD and other contraceptive users.[87,88] Among infertile women, hysterosalpingogram or laparoscopic evidence of prior tubal infection was related to *C. trachomatis* antibody and the prior use of an IUD.[89] A further increase in the rate of tubal damage was observed in patients with *C. trachomatis* antibody and prior IUD use.[89] Prior *C. trachomatis* infection and prior IUD use were independently related to tubal damage.

The IUD also causes focal necrosis of the endometrium at the point of attachment leading to breaks in the endometrial barrier.[90] Plasma cells are typically present in the endometrium and in the fallopian tubes of 50% of women wearing an IUD.[91] Plasma cells typically migrate into this tissue in response to the presence of a foreign antigen. The inflammatory response that was attributed to the foreign body effect of the IUD is instead in response to the bacterial antigen present on the IUD. This response may adversely influence the ability of the tissue to protect itself from infection.

As expected, IUD use is associated with an increased rate of tubal infertility. Primary tubal infertility was increased twofold[34,69] in IUD users compared to those not using contraception or other contraception. Infertility tended to be higher for Dalkon Shield than other IUD users, but among those who used only one IUD in their lifetime, copper devices were associated with a significant 1.6[69] to 3.1[75] increased risk of tubal infertility. Multivariate adjustment was made for confounding variables identified in the studies. Progesterone containing IUDs may have a lower PID rate than copper IUDs, perhaps related to an effect similar to that of oral contraceptives in reducing the rate of chlamydial PID. Infertile patients who had a history of gonorrhea or PID had higher relative risks of infertility than those without, but the effect of the IUD on infertility was independent of whether the patient had a prior episode of gonorrhea or PID.[69]

Human Immunodeficiency Virus

Recent reports indicated that women with PID have a higher frequency of human immunodeficiency virus (HIV) infection than observed in other gynecologic practice settings.[92-94] Human immunodeficiency virus infection is related to drug use which, in turn is related to cervical infection. Thus, drug use may confound the relationship.[94] On the other hand, patients with decreased immunity may have an increased rate of acquiring infection. In addition, patients with HIV infection have reactivation of latent infections such as tuberculosis, cytomegalovirus and toxoplasmosis, and it is possible that HIV infection causes reactivation of chlamydia, a phenomenon previously proposed.[57]

References

1. Aral SO, Mosher WD, Cates W Jr. Self-reported pelvic inflammatory disease in the United States, 1988. *JAMA* 1991;**266**:2570–2573.
2. Expert Committee on Pelvic Inflammatory Disease. Pelvic inflammatory disease: Research directions in the 1990s. *Sex Trans Dis* 1991;**18**:46–64.
3. Weström L. Incidence, prevalence, and trends of acute pelvic inflammatory disease and its consequences in industrialized countries. *Am J Obstet Gynecol* 1980;**138**:880–892.
4. Cates W Jr. Sexually transmitted disease, pelvic inflammatory disease, and infertility: An epidemiologic update. *Epidemiol Rev* 1990;**12**:199–220.
5. Washington AE, Aral SO, Wølner-Hanssen P, Grimes DA, Holmes KK. Assessing risk for pelvic inflammatory disease and its sequelae. *JAMA* 1991;**266**:2581–2586.
6. Lee NC, Rubin GL, Grimes DA. Measures of sexual behavior and the risk of pelvic inflammatory disease. *Obstet Gynecol* 1991;**77**:425–430.
7. Brown IM, Cruikshank JG. Aetiology factors in pelvic inflammatory disease in urban blacks in Rhodesia. *S Afr Med J* 1976;**50**:1342–1344.
8. Eschenbach DA, Harnish JP, Holmes KK. Pathogenesis of acute pelvic inflammatory disease: Role of contraception and other risk factors. *Am J Obstet Gynecol* 1977;**128**:838–850.
9. Forslin L, Falk V, Danielsson D. Changes in the incidence of acute gonococcal and nongonococcal salpingitis. *Br J Vener Dis* 1978;**54**:247.
10. Rees E, Annels EH. Gonococcal salpingitis. *Br J Vener Dis* 1969;**45**:205–210.
11. McCormack WM, Stumacher RJ, Johnson K, et al. A clinical spectrum of gonococcal infection in women. *Lancet* 1977;**1**:1182–1186.
12. Copplson M, Pixley E, Reid B. *Colposcopy*. Springfield, IL, Charles C. Thomas, Publisher, 1971.
13. Ayra OP, Mallinson H, Goddard AO. Epidemiological and clinical correlates of chlamydial infection of the cervix. *Br J Vener Dis* 1981;**57**:118–124.
14. Hobson D, Karayiannis P, Byng RE, Rees E, Tait IA, Davies JA. Quantitative aspects of chlamydial infection of the cervix. *Br J Vener Dis* 1980;**56**:156–162.
15. Enhorning G, Huldt L, Melen B. Ability of cervical mucus to act as a barrier against bacteria. *Am J Obstet Gynecol* 1970;**108**:532–537.
16. Buchanan TM, Eschenbach DA, Knapp JS, Holmes KK. Gonococcal salpingitis is less likely to recur with *Neisseria gonorrheae* of the same prinicipal outer membrane antigenic type. *Am J Obstet Gynecol* 1980;**138**:978–980.
17. Bell TA, Holmes KK. Age-specific risks of syphilis, gonorrhea, and hospitalized pelvic inflammatory disease in sexually experienced U.S. women. *Sex Trans Dis* 1984;**11**:291–295.
18. Washington AE, Sweet RL, Shafer M-A. Pelvic inflammatory disease and its sequelae in adolescents. *J Adolesc Health Care* 1985;**6**:298–310.
19. Eschenbach DA, Stevens C, Critchlow C, Holmes KK. Epidemiology of acute pelvic inflammatory disease. Abstract #C-03-088 presented at the International Society of STD Research, October 6–9, 1991, Banff, Canada.
20. D'Costa LJ, et al. Prostitutes are a major reservoir of sexually transmitted disease in Nairobi, Kenya. *Sex Transm Dis* 1985;**12**:64–69.

21. Handsfield HH, et al. Criteria for selective screening for Chlamydia trachomatis infection in women attending family planning clinics. *JAMA* 1986;**255**:1730–1735.

22. Schachter J, Stoner E, Moncada J. Screening for chlamydial infections in women attending family planning clinics. *West J Med* 1983;**138**:375–379.

23. Flesh G, Weiner JM, Corlett RC Jr, et al. The intrauterine device and acute salpingitis: A multifactor analysis. *Am J Obstet Gynecol* 1979;**135**:402–408.

24. Wølner-Hanssen P, Eschenbach DA, Paavonen J, et al. Decreased risk of symptomatic chlamydial pelvic inflammatory disease associated with oral contraceptive use. *JAMA* 1990;**263**:54–59.

25. Lidegaard O, Helm P. Pelvic infammatory disease: The influence of contraceptive, sexual, and social life events. Contraception 1990;**41**:475–483.

26. Toth A, O'Leary WM, Ledger WJ. Evidence for microbial transfer by the spermatozoa. *Obstet Gynecol* 1982;**59**:556–559.

27. Friberg J, Confino E, Suarez M, et al. *Chlamydia trachomatis* attached to spermatozoa recovered from the peritoneal cavity of patients with salpingitis. *J Reprod Med* 1987;**32**:120–122.

28. Cunningham FG, Hauth JC, Strong JD, et al. Evaluation of tetracycline or penicillin and ampicillin for treatment of acute pelvic inflammatory disease. *N Engl J Med* 1977;**296**:1380–1386.

29. Eschenbach DA, Buchanan TM, Pollock HM, et al. Polymicrobial etiology of acute pelvic inflammatory disease. *N Engl J Med* 1975;**293**:166–171.

30. Darrow WW, Kiegel K. Preventive health behavior and STD, in Holmes KK, Mardh P-A, Sparling PF, Wiesner PJ (eds): *Sexually Transmitted Diseases*, 2nd ed. New York, McGraw-Hill Information Services Co, 1990, pp 85–92.

31. Wølner-Hanssen P, Kiviat NB, Holmes KK. Atypical pelvic inflammatory disease: Subacute, chronic or subclinical upper genital tract infection in women, in Holmes KK, Mardh P-A, Sparling PF, Wiesner PJ (eds): *Sexually Transmitted Diseases*, 2nd ed. New York, McGraw-Hill Information Services Co, 1990, pp 615–620.

32. Marchbanks PA, Lee NC, Peterson HB. Cigarette smoking as a risk factor for pelvic inflammatory disease. *Am J Obstet Gynecol* 1990;**162**:639–644.

33. Phipps WR, Cramer DW, Schiff I, et al. The association between smoking and female infertility as influenced by cause of the infertility. *Fertil Steril* 1987;**48**:377–382.

34. Daling JR, Weiss NS, Metch BJ, Chow WH, Soderstrom RM, Moore DE, Spadoni LR, Stadel BV. Primary tubal infertility in relation to the use of an intrauterine device. *N Engl J Med* 1985;**312**:937–941.

35. Chow W-H, Daling JR, Weiss NS, et al. Maternal cigarette smoking and tubal pregnancy. *Obstet Gynecol* 1988;**71**:167–170.

36. Sasson JM, Haley NJ, Hoffman D, Wynder EL, Hellborn D, Nilsson S. Cigarette smoking and neoplasia of the uterine cervix: Smoke consituents in cervical mucus. *N Engl J Med* 1985;**312**:315–319.

37. Neri A, Eskerling B. Influence of smoking and adrenaline (epinephrine) on the uterotubal insufflation test (Rubin test). *Fertil Steril* 1969;**20**:818–828.

38. Phillips B, Marshall E, Brown S, et al. Effect of smoking on human natural killer cell activity. *Cancer* 1985;**56**:2789–2792.

39. Hersey P, Prendergast D, Edwards A. Effects of cigarette smoking on the immune system: Follow-up studies in normal subjects after cessation of smoking. *Med J Aust* 1983;**2**:425–429.

40. Halsey NS, Coberly JS, Holt E, Coreil J, Kissinger P, Moulton LH, Brutus J-R, Boulos R. Sexual behavior, smoking, and HIV-1 infection in Haitian women. *JAMA* 1992;**267**:2062–2066.

41. Baron JA, LaVecchia C, Levi F. The antiestrogen effect of cigarette smoking in women. *Am J Obstet Gynecol* 1990;**162**:502–514.

42. Rank RG, White HJ, Hough AJ Jr., et al. Effect of estradiol on chlamydial genital infection of female guinea pigs. *Infect Immun* 1982;**38**:699–705.

43. Pasley JN, Rank RG, Hough AJ Jr., et al. Effects of various doses of estradiol on chlamydia genital infection in ovariectomized guinea pigs. *Sex Transm Dis* 1985;**12**:8–13.

44. Forrest KA, Washington AE, Daling JR, et al. Vaginal douching as a possible risk factor for pelvic inflammatory disease. *J Natl Med Assoc* 1989;**81**: 159–165.

45. Limsuwan A, Vachrotai S, Panupornprapong Y, et al. A clinical trial of a vaginal preparation regimen for the prophylaxis of gonorrhea. *J Med Assoc Thai* 1978;**61**:485–490.

46. Neumann HH, DeCherney A. Douching and pelvic inflammatory disease. *N Engl J Med* 1976;**295**:789.

47. Wølner-Hanssen P, Eschenbach DA, Paavonen J, et al. Association between vaginal douching and acute pelvic inflammatory disease. *JAMA* 1990;**263**:1936–1941.

48. Chow WH, Daling JR, Weiss NS, et al. Vaginal douching as a potential risk factor for tubal ectopic pregnancy. *Am J Obstet Gynecol* 1985;**153**:727–729.

49. Falk V, Krook G. Do results of culture for gonococci vary with the sampling phase of menstrual cycle? *Acta Derm Venereol* 1967;**47**:190–195.

50. Sweet RL, Blankfort-Doyle M, Robbie MO, et al. The occurrence of chlamydial and gonococcal salpingitis during the menstrual cycle. *JAMA* 1986;**255**:2062–2064.

51. Draper DC, James JF, Brooks GF, et al. Comparison of virulence markers of peritoneal and fallopian tube isolates with endocervical *N. gonorrhoeae* isolates from women with acute salpingitis. *Infect Immun* 1980;**27**:882–890.

52. Weström L. Effect of acute pelvic inflammatory disease on fertility. *Am J Obstet Gynecol* 1975;**121**:707–713.

53. Patton DL, Moore DE, Spadoni LR, Soules MR, Halber SA, Wang S-P. A comparison of the fallopian tube's responses to overt and silent salpingitis. *Obstet Gynecol* 1989;**73**:622–630.

54. Patton DL, Kuo CC, Wang SP, Halber SA. Distal tubal obstruction induced by repeated *Chlamydia trachomatis* salpingeal infections in pig-tailed macaques. *J Infect Dis* 1987;**155**:1292–1299.

55. Brooks GF, Darrow WW, Day JA. Repeated gonorrhea: An analysis of importance and risk factors. *J Infect Dis* 1978;**137**:161–169.

56. Patton DL, Wølner-Hanssen P, Cosgrove SJ, Holmes KK. The effects of *Chlamydia trachomatis* on the female reproductive tract of the *Macaca nemestrina* after a single tubal challenge following repeated cervical inoculations. *Obstet Gynecol* 1990;**76**:643–650.

57. Betteiger BE, Fraiz J, Newhall WJ, Katz BP, Jones RB. Association of recurrent chlamydial infection with gonorrhea. *J Infect Dis* 1989;**159**:661–669.
58. Austin A, Louv WC, Alexander J. A case-control study of spermicides and gonorrhea. *JAMA* 1984;**251**:2822–2824.
59. Quinn RW, O'Reilly KR. Contraceptive practices of women attending the sexually transmitted disease clinic in Nashville, Tennessee. *Sex Trans Dis* 1985;**12**:99–102.
60. Louv WC, Austin H, Alexander WJ, Stagno S, Cheeks J. A clinical trial of nonoxynol-9 for preventing gonococcal and chlamydial infections. *J Infec Dis* 1988;**158**:518–523.
61. Kelaghan J, Rubin GL, Ory HW, Layde PM. Barrier-method contraceptives and pelvic inflammatory disease. *JAMA* 1982;**248**:184–187.
62. Harrison HR, Costin M, Meder JB, Bownds SM, Sim DA, Lewis M, Alexander ER. Cervical *Chlamydia trachomatis* infection in university women: Relationship to history, contraception, ectopy and cervicitis. *Am J Obstet Gynecol* 1985;**153**;244–251.
63. Cromer A, Heald FP. Pelvic inflammatory disease associated with *Neisseria gonorrhoeae* and *Chlamydia trachomatis*: Clinical correlates. *Sex Trans Dis* 1987;**14**:125–129.
64. Weström L, Bengtsson L-P, Mardh P-A. The risk of pelvic inflammatory disease in women using intrauterine contraceptive devices as compared to nonusers. *Lancet* 1976;**2**:221–224.
65. Wølner-Hanssen P, Svensson L, Mardh P-A, Weström L. Laparsoceopic findings and contraceptive use in women with signs and symptoms suggestive of acute salpingitis. *Obstet Gynecol* 1986;**66**:233–238.
66. Svensson L, Weström L, Mardh P-A. Contraceptives and acute salpingitis. *JAMA* 1984;**251**:2553–2555.
67. Kinghorn GR, Waugh MA. Oral contraceptive use and prevalence of infection with *Chlamydia trachomatis* in women. *Br J Vener Dis* 1981;**57**:187–190.
68. Ryden G, Fahrseus L, Molin L, Ahman K. Do contraceptives influence the incidence of acute pelvic inflammatory disease in women with gonorrhea? *Contraception* 1979;**20**:149–157.
69. Cramer DW, Schiff I, Schoenbaum SC, Gibson M, Belisle S, Albrecht B, Stillman RJ, Berger MJ, Wilson E, Stadel BV, Seibel M. Tubal infertility and the intrauterine device. *N Engl J Med* 1985;**312**:941–947.
70. Senanayake P, Kramer DG. Contraception and the etiology of pelvic inflammatory disease: New perspectives. *Am J Obstet Gynecol* 1980;**138**:852–860.
71. Lee NC, Rubin GL, Ory HW, Burkman RT. Type of intrauterine device and the risk of pelvic inflammatory disease. *Obstet Gynecol* 1983;**62**:1–6.
72. Sparks H, Purrier BGA, Watt PJ, Elstein M. Bacteriological colonisation of uterine cavity; Role of tailed intrauterine contraceptive device. *Brit Med J* 1981;**282**:1189–1191.
73. Valicenti JF, Pappas AA, Graber CD, Williamson HO, Fowler Willis N. Detection and prevalence of IUD-associated *Actinomyces* colonization and related morbidity: A prospective study of 69,925 cervical smears. *JAMA* 1982;**247**:1149–1152.
74. Marrie TJ, Costerton JW. A scanning and transmission electron microscopic study of the surfaces of intrauterine contraceptive devices. *Am J Obstet Gynecol* 1983;**146**:384–394.

75. Daling JR, Weiss NS, Voight LF, McKnight B, Moore DE. The intrauterine device and primary tubal infertility. *N Engl J Med* 1992;**326**:203–204.
76. Grimes DA. Intrauterine devices and pelvic inflammatory disease: Recent developments. *Contraception* 1987;**36**:97–109.
77. Vessey MP, Doll R, Peto R, et al. A long term follow-up study of women using different methods of contraception-An interim report. *J Biosoc Sci* 1976;**8**: 373–426.
78. Kessel E. Pelvic inflammatory disease with intrauterine device use: A reassessment. *Fertil Steril* 1989;**51**:1–11.
79. Mishell DR, Moyer DL. Association of pelvic inflammatory disease with the intrauterine device. *Clin Obstet Gynecol* 1969;**12**:179–197.
80. Tietze C, Lewit S. Evaluation of intrauterine devices: Ninth progress report of the cooperative statistical program. *Stud Fam Plann* 1970;**55**:537–576.
81. Marrie TJ, Costerton JW. A scanning and transmission electron microscopic study of the surfaces of intrauterine contraceptive devices. *Am J Obstet Gynecol* 1983;**146**:384–394.
82. Haukkamaa M, Stranden P, Jousimies-Somer H, Siitonen A. Bacterial flora of the cervix in women using different methods of contraception. *Am J Obstet Gynecol* 1986;**154**:520–524.
83. Haukkamaa M, Stranden P, Jousimies-Somer H, Siitonen A. Bacterial flora of the cervix in women using an intrauterine device. *Contraception* 1987;**36**: 527–534.
84. Hill JA, Talledo E, Steele J. Quantitative transcervical uterine cultures in asymptomatic women using an intrauterine contraceptive device. *Obstet Gynecol* 1986;**68**:700–704.
85. Noonan AS, Adams JB. Gonorrhea screening in an urban hospital family planning program. *Am J Public Health* 1974;**64**:700–704.
86. Berger GS, Keith L, Moss W. Prevalence of gonorrhoea among women using various methods of contraception. *Brit J Vener Dis* 1975;**51**:307–309.
87. Gjonnaess H, Dalaker K, Anestad G, Mardh P-A, Kvile G, Bergan T. Pelvic inflammatory disease: Etiologic studies with emphasis on chlamydial infection. *Obstet Gynecol* 1982;**59**:550–555.
88. Osser S, Persson K. Epidemiologic and serodiagnostic aspects of chlamydial salpingitis. *Obstet Gynecol* 1982;**59**:206–209.
89. Gump DW, Gibson M, Ashikaga T. Evidence of prior pelvic inflammatory disease and its relationship to *Chlamydia trachomatis* antibody and intrauterine contraceptive device use in infertile women. *Am J Obstet Gynecol* 1983;**146**: 153–159.
90. Shepard BL, Bonnar J. The effects of intrauterine contraceptive devices on the ultrastructure of the endometrium in relation to bleeding complications. *Am J Obstet Gynecol* 1983;**146**:829–839.
91. Beerthuizen RJCM, Van Wijck JAM, Eskes TKAB, Vermeulen AHM, Vooijs GP. IUD and salpingitis: A prospective study of pathomorphological changes in the oviducts in IUD-users. *Europ J Obstet Gynecol Reprod Biol* 1982;**13**: 31–41.
92. Hoegsberg B, Abulafia O, Sedlis A, Feldman J, Desjalais D, Landesman S, Minkoff H. Sexually transmitted diseases and human immunodeficiency virus infection among women with pelvic inflammatory disease. *Am J Obstet Gynecol* 1990;**163**:1135–1139.

93. Sperling RS, Friedman F Jr, Joyner M, Brodman M, Dottino P. Seroprevalence of human immunodeficiency virus in women admitted to the hospital with pelvic inflammatory disease. *J Reprod Med* 1991;**36**:122–124.

94. Safrin S, Dattel BJ, Hauer L, Sweet RL. Seroprevalence and epidemiologic correlates of human immunodeficiency virus infection in women with acute pelvic inflammatory disease. *Obstet Gynecol* 1990;**75**:666–670.

2
Risk Factors for Pelvic Inflammatory Disease and Associated Sequelae

NANCY S. PADIAN AND A. EUGENE WASHINGTON

Unlike an infectious disease associated with the presence of a particular etiologic agent, pelvic inflammatory disease (PID) is a syndrome or constellation of symptoms that can result from multiple etiologic pathways. Approximately 75% of PID is associated with progression of an initial infection from various sexually transmitted disease (STD) pathogens in the lower genital tract into the upper genital tract.[1] In cases of PID not associated with an initial STD, the initial exposure may involve a mechanical insult (e.g., traumatic birth, abortion, and IUD insertion) that may result in a perturbation of the normal flora of the vagina, or a disruption such that the normal flora of the lower genital tract flora ascends into the endometrial cavity or fallopian tubes.[2] Of course it is possible that this pathogenic mechanism may also occur from disturbances caused by STD infections.[2]

A natural history time line from initial exposure to an STD pathogen to development of PID (systemic or invasive disease) and then the occurrence of PID-associated sequelae is depicted in Figure 2.1. The initial exposure most likely would be (but is not limited) to *Chlamydia trachomatis* (CT) or *Neisseria gonorrhoeae* (GC). As portrayed on the time line, infection associated with these pathogens can result in disease that may or may not be symptomatic. For example, chlamydial infections can result in symptomatic cervicitis in women or urethritis in men, or in asymptomatic infections involving these sites. The presence of symptoms is not necessary for disease to progress to PID that itself may not be clinically apparent. In PID cases not believed to be sexually transmitted, invasive disease could result directly from exposure or initial insult without initial STD infection as an intermediary step. Finally, PID (regardless of its etiology), may progress to adverse long-term sequelae (e.g., infertility, ectopic pregnancy, chronic pelvic pain, pelvic adhesions, and other inflammatory residua that may require surgical intervention).[3]

Because the vast majority of PID is believed to be sexually transmitted, the rest of this chapter will focus on this etiology, and risk factors will be

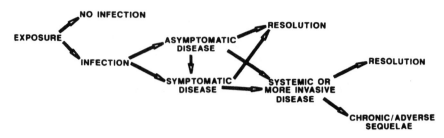

FIGURE 2.1. Natural history time line.

identified at each step along the time line.[4,5] Table 2.1 provides a delineation of risk factors associated with STD acquisition, the development of PID, and the development of PID sequelae.[5] What follows is an overview of risk factors unique to each of these disease processes.

TABLE 2.1. Health outcome affected.

Risk variable	Acquisition of STD	Development of PID	Development of PID sequelae
Demographic/social indicators			
Age	+	+	−
Socioeconomic status	+	+	•
Marital status	+	+	•
Residence, rural/urban	+	•	•
Individual behavior/practices			
Sexual behavior			
Number of partners	+	•	•
Age at first sexual intercourse	+	•	•
Frequency of sexual intercourse	+	•	•
Rate of acquiring new partners	+	•	•
Contraceptive practice			
Barrier	−	−	−
Pills	+	−	•
Intrauterine device	•	+	+
Health-care behavior			
Evaluation of symptoms	+	+	+
Compliance with treatment instructions	+	+	+
Sex partner referral	+	+	+
Others			
Douching	•	+	•
Smoking	+	+	•
Substance abuse	+	•	•
Menstrual cycle	+	+	•

STD = sexually transmitted diseases; PID = pelvic inflammatory disease.
Variable may be associated with increased risk (+) or decreased risk (−), or no association reported (•).

Risk Factors Associated with Acquisition of an Initial STD Infection

Risk factors associated with exposure to an infection from STD pathogens may or may not be associated with progression of lower genital tract infection to the upper genital tract. Table 2.2 lists the categories of risk factors associated with STD transmission. Specific risk factors that are associated with STD acquisition in Table 2.1 are encompassed by the parameters in Table 2.2. The four major categories of risk factors that effect STD spread are: (1) selection and characteristics of the sex partner, (2) infectivity and susceptibility, (3) duration of infection, and (4) sociocultural context in which sexual behavior occurs.[6] These parameters were derived from models of the transmission dynamics of STDs that are based on the following equation:[7] $R = BDC$, where R is the secondary infection rate (the rate of incident infection from a primary case), B represents the transmission coefficient (infectivity plus susceptibility), D represents the length of the infectious period, and C represents the mean rate of partner change.

Sex Partner Selection and Characteristics

The most obvious risk factor related to sex partner selection is the number of partners. Larger numbers of partners increases the chance that at least one partner is infected. However, the probability that any one partner is

TABLE 2.2. Categories of risk factors associated with STD transmission.

1. Sex partner characteristics
   Number of partners
   Probability that partner is infected
      Prevalence of infection
      Patterns of partner selection
2. Infectivity rates
   Infectiousness
      Size of inoculum
      Timing of pathogen shedding
   Susceptibility
      Genetic factors
      Immunological factors
      Coinfection with other organisms
      Anatomical features
   Behavioral factors
      Types of sexual and contraceptive practices
      Hygienic practices
      Substance abuse
3. Duration of infection
4. Sociocultural environment

infected is also associated with the prevalence of infection within the community from which the partner was selected. For example, having large numbers of partners in an area with a low prevalence of infection may not result in selection of an infected partner, whereas if the prevalence of infection were high, it may only take a few partners to select one that is infected. Partner characteristics (the behavioral profile of a partner as well as how, when, and where partners are selected) also contribute to the probability that a partner is infected. These characteristics include whether the partner had other partners who were infected, whether the partner uses drugs, the setting in which partners meet (e.g., park, school, or bar), and the validity of reliable partner histories (if elicited).[6]

Infectivity and Susceptibility

Once exposed, transmission does not necessarily occur. The infectivity rate (probability that transmission will occur after one exposure) of various pathogens differ. For example, it is more difficult to transmit human immunodeficiency virus (HIV) than GC, all other factors being equal. However, all exposures are not equal, and several biological factors mediate infectivity rates. Infectiousness may vary according to the amount of infectious dose or a particular pathogenic strain. Susceptibility in the exposed partner also effects transmission probabilities and includes genetic factors, immunological status, coinfection with other organisms, nonspecific defense mechanisms such as those related to normal flora, and anatomical features due to age.[6]

Behavioral risk factors that affect infectiousness and susceptibility and thus the probability of transmission also have been identified.[5,6] These include specific sexual practices such as number of sexual contacts (which increases the likelihood that any one contact will result in transmission), anal intercourse, sexual intercourse during menstruation, and lack of barrier contraceptive practices, particularly condoms. Behavioral factors also include substance abuse, mainly during intercourse (because of the association between drug or alcohol use and failure to use barrier contraceptives). Hygienic practices such as lack of circumcision, tampon use, and smoking all have been associated with STD acquisition.

Biological and behavioral factors may account for the apparent increased risk of STD acquisition among individuals of young age.[4,5] Young women ≤20 years of age have a larger zone of ectopy and greater penetrability of cervical mucus, both of which are correlated with STD acquisition. These same young women, particularly those who begin sexual activity during their early teen years, also tend to have large numbers of sex partners.

Duration of Infection

The duration of infection refers to the amount of time an infectious organism is viable in the host before it is eliminated by the natural resolution of infection.[6] Duration of infection is important because the longer an infection persists, the longer an infected individual is able to transmit infection to susceptible partners, thus increasing the prevalence of infection within a community. Estimates of the duration of infection may include effects of treatment of specific immune functions. Furthermore, sometimes an infection may be asymptomatic and may go unrecognized and thus persist for a longer time prior to treatment. In addition, asymptomatic individuals, by definition, do not appear sick and are thus unlikely to be perceived by partners as infected. This explains why transmission from asymptomatic individuals is often thought to be the driving force behind epidemic spread of infectious disease agents.[8]

The duration of infectiousness does not exactly correlate with the duration of infection because an infected individual does not necessarily shed the infectious pathogen in a uniform manner. Pathogens may be shed (and thus be infectious) transiently (as in hepatitis B infection), intermittently (as in herpes simplex virus infection or infection with HIV), or at various points during the natural history of infection.

Sociocultural Context

The sociocultural milieu in which sexual behavior occurs also affects the likelihood of transmission, although in an indirect fashion.[6] Likelihood that condoms will be used or acceptance of sexual contact with prostitutes varies by culture. Similarly, political and economic factors such as political changes, war, or economic reforms may result in concomitant social reorganization that affect norms of sexual behavior. Biotechnological developments such as advances in treatment of development and distribution of contraceptives also affect acceptable sexual behaviors and thus the likelihood of transmission. Other social factors such as availability of health care, access to treatment, and level of social disorganization that result from impoverished living conditions undoubtedly contribute to overrepresentation of minority races among individuals infected with STDs.

Risk Factors Associated with Development of PID

As is apparent in Table 2.1, several risk factors are associated with acquisition of an initial STD and development of PID.[5] These factors include young age, lack of barrier contraceptives, substance abuse, and smoking. Factors associated with transmission delineated in Table 2.2 are also associated with progression. For example, the longer the duration of an untreated infection, the greater the likelihood that infection will spread to other anatomical sites, thereby increasing the severity of disease and the likelihood of the development of invasive disease.[6] Because these factors are associated with two outcomes on the time line (STD acquisition as well as the development of PID), it is difficult to identify those factors independently associated with the development of PID. Identification of risk factors unique to the development of PID may elucidate the pathogenic mechanism by which infection ascends to the upper genital tract, thus initiating the development of PID. Three risk factors have been identified that appear to be uniquely associated with the development of PID[5]: oral contraceptive (OC) use, douching, and use of an intrauterine device (IUD).

The mechanism by which OCs contribute to the development of PID is not completely understood.[9] On the one hand, use of OCs seems to facilitate CT infection in the endocervix, although the role of OCs in facilitating initial acquisition of GC remains unclear.[10] Most likely, OC use increases the zone of ectopy, revealing a greater area of columnar epithelium, target cells for CT. However, CT may simply be easier to culture among women who are OC users, resulting in a detection bias rather than an elevated infection rate. On the other hand, there appears to be a protective effect of OC use on PID development among women with an initial CT infection.[10,11] This means that although OCs may increase the likelihood of acquisition to an STD, they may decrease the likelihood of progression of infection to the upper genital tract once a women has an initial CT infection. Two hypotheses have been postulated to explain such a protective mechanism[5]: increased cervical mucus that prevents ascension of infection and decreased menstrual blood that provides fertile growth media for infection. However, it remains speculative even among women with CT, whether OC use actually prevents ascension of infection into the fallopian tubes or whether they simply protect against symptomatic infection.

Douching and IUD use may be seen as mechanical insults that facilitate ascension of normal and abnormal flora from the vagina and cervix into the upper genital tract. Douching may flush vaginal and cervical microorganisms into the upper genital tract.[12,13] Thus, pathogens responsible for initial lower genital tract infections may be introduced into the upper genital tract through the mechanics of douching. Alternatively, douching may flush away normally protective vaginal flora, thus reducing competition among naturally occurring organisms that could then permit the growth of bacteria.[5] If this latter hypothesis was true, douching should also increase initial acquisition of an initial STD, whereas to date, douching has only been observed as a risk factor for PID and other long-term sequelae such as ectopic pregnancies.[14] A final hypothesis proposes that douching introduces the presentation of normal flora of the vagina and cervix into the upper genital tract, resulting initially in bacterial vaginosis and ultimately in PID.[2,15]

One interesting study has correlated douching with STD risks or symptomatology.[16] The hypothesis here is that douching could be associated with ascension of infection because it is indirectly associated with initial acquisition of an STD: symptomatic and thus infected women were simply more likely to douche. Because multivariate analyses that separate the effects of douching from STD infection were not conducted, further study needs to be done in this area.

IUDs represent a physical mechanism that can introduce either bacterial infection from the lower genital tract or endogenous vaginal or cervical organisms into the uterus during their insertion.[4,17,18] This theory has been supported by studies that show increased risk associated with IUD insertion only within the first 20 days after their insertion.[19] After this time, there is less opportunity for ascension of organisms. In addition, studies that have examined IUD use show increased risk mainly among those women who live in areas with high background rates of STDs.[19] This could explain the association between IUD use and PID among women with high-risk sexual behavior (e.g., large number of partners): such behavior is a marker for current STD infection. This theory is supported by studies that demonstrate decreased risk of PID after IUD insertion among women who were given prophylactic doxycycline hyclate at the time of insertion.[20] Multisite clinical trials are underway to further examine this phenomenon.

Risk Factors Associated with Development of PID-Associated Sequelae

Less is known about unique risk factors associated with PID sequelae than about risk factors associated with STD acquisition and development of PID subsequent to an initial STD infection. As delineated in Table 2.1, several risk factors associated with the development of PID may also be associated with the development of sequelae. These factors include the duration of disease, determined, in part, of the time from diagnosis and evaluation of symptoms to initiation of treatment, douching, smoking, and method of contraception. Most of these factors are discussed above. For example, there is some evidence that use of an IUD and smoking may contribute to subsequent infertility,[4,5] but it is unclear whether these factors are independently related to infertility. The link with infertility could be indirect and may result from their association with PID that is associated with infertility and not smoking or IUD use per se.

An inverse association may exist between PID-associated sequelae and young age.[4] Although young age is associated with acquisition of an initial STD infection and increased probability of the development of PID, available data suggest that young age may also be associated with a decreased likelihood of adverse long-term sequelae after an initial PID mechanism. However, studies that have examined the effect of age have been cross-sectional. Although older women may have higher rates of long-term sequelae, they also may have had repeat STD infections (or long-term asymptomatic infections) or repeat episodes of PID (also including the possibility of asymptomatic and undiagnosed tubal infection) prior to the initiation of the study. Prospective studies that follow the same groups of women over time are necessary to elucidate the true association between age and sequelae.

Repeat episodes of PID are the most well-established risk factor for long-term sequelae.[4] Repeat episodes are associated with an increased likelihood of permanent damage and concomitant irreversible long-term sequelae. For example, tubal factor infertility had been estimated to occur among 13% to 40% of all women who have experienced at least one episode of PID.[3,4,21,22] This percentage increases dramatically with repeat episodes of PID, and may be as high as 75% among those women who have had three PID episodes.[4]

Clinician's Behavior/Practices as Risk Factors

Failure to assess a woman's risk of PID, make a timely diagnosis, and provide appropriate treatment may be viewed as a risk factor for increased acquisition of STD, development of PID, and development of PID sequelae. Practitioners can influence a woman's risk of infection by providing effective counseling about their sexual behavior and health-care practices (e.g., douching, smoking, and substance abuse), and by convincing them to comply with management instructions. Timely diagnosis and appropriate treatment of lower genital tract chlamydial and gonococcal infections and subsequent PID can reduce risk of adverse consequences in the infected individual and risk of further transmission to others. By also ensuring timely and effective treatment of women's sex partners, practitioners can reduce risk of reinfection.[23] Moreover, because a sex partner's infection may be asymptomatic, treating the partner may reduce risk for development of complications as well as further transmission of infection. Although specific evidence supporting the efficacy of these clinical practices[24] is scarce, neglecting to apply them consistently may indeed place a woman at increased risk for infection and disease.

References

1. Rice PA, Schachter J. Pathogenesis of pelvic inflammatory diseases. *JAMA* 1991;**266**:2587–2594.
2. Wasserheit J. Pelvic inflammatory disease and infertility. *Md Med J* 1987;**36**: 58–63.
3. Pearce M. Pelvic inflammatory disease. *BMJ* 1990;**300**:1090–1091.
4. Cates W, Rolfs R, Aral S. Sexually transmitted diseases, pelvic inflammatory disease, and infertility: An epidemiologic update. *Epidemiol Rev* 1990;**12**: 199–220.
5. Washington AE, Aral S, Wølner-Hanssen P, et al. Assessing risk for pelvic inflammatory disease and its sequelae. *JAMA* 1991;**266**:2581–2586.
6. Padian N, Shiboski S, Hitchcock P. Risk factors for acquisition of sexually transmitted diseases and development of complications, in Wasserheit J, Aral S,

Holmes K, Hitchcock P, (eds): *Research Issues in Human Behavior and Sexually Transmitted Diseases in the AIDS Era*. Washington, DC. Am. Soc. Microbiology 1991, pp 83–96.

7. May R, Anderson R. Transmission dynamics of HIV infection. *Nature* 1987;**326**:137–142.
8. Lilienfeld A, Lilienfeld D. Foundations of Epidemiology. New York, Oxford University Press, 1980.
9. Washington AE, Gove S, Schachter J, et al. Oral contraceptives, *Chlamydia trachomatis* infection and pelvic inflammatory disease: A word of caution about protection. *JAMA* 1985;**253**:2246–2250.
10. Wølner-Hanssen P, Eschenbach DA, Paavonen J, et al. Decreased risk of symptomatic chlamydial pelvic inflammatory disease associated with oral contraceptive use. *JAMA* 1990;**263**:54–59.
11. Senanayake P, Kramer D. Contraception and the etiology of pelvic inflammatory disease: New perspectives. *Am J Obstet Gynecol* 1980;**138**:852–860.
12. McGowan L. Peritonitis following the vaginal douche and a proposed alternative method for vaginal and vulvar care. *Am J Obstet Gynecol* 1965;**93**:506–509.
13. Egenolf G, McNaughton R. Chemical peritonitis resulting from vaginal douche: Report of a case. *Obstet Gynecol* 1956;**7**:23–24.
14. Chow J, Yonekura L, Richwald G, et al. The association between *Chlamydia trachomatis* and ectopic pregnancy: A matched-pair, case-control study. *JAMA* 1990;**263**:3164–3167.
15. Wølner-Hanssen P, Eschenbach D, Paavonen J, et al. Association between vaginal douching and acute pelvic inflammatory disease. *JAMA* 1990;**263**:1936–1941.
16. Rosenberg MJ, Phillips RS, Holmes MD. Vaginal douching: Who and why? *J Reprod Med* 1991;**36**(10):753–758.
17. Lee NC, Rubin G, Ory H, et al. Type of intrauterine device and the risk of pelvic inflammatory disease. *Obstet Gynecol* 1983;**62**:1–6.
18. Grimes D. Intrauterine devices and pelvic inflammatory disease: Recent developments. *Contraception* 1987;**36**:97–109.
19. Farley T, Rosenberg M, Rowe P, et al. Intrauterine devices and pelvic inflammatory disease: An international perspective. *Lancet* 1992;**1**:785–788.
20. Sinei S, Schulz K, Lamptey P, et al. Preventing IUCD-related pelvic infection: The efficacy of prophylactic doxycycline at insertion. *Br J Obstet Gynaecol* 1990;**97**:412–419.
21. Westr
öm L. Affect of acute pelvic inflammatory disease on fertility. *Am J Obstet Gynecol* 1975;**121**:707–713.
22. Weström L. Introductory address: Treatment of pelvic inflammatory disease in view of etiology and risk factors. *Sex Trans Dis* 1984;**11**:437–440.
23. Katz B, Danos C, Quinn T, et al. Efficiency and cost-effectiveness of field follow-up for patients with *Chlamydia trachomatis* infection in a sexually transmitted disease clinic. *Sex Trans Dis* 1988;**15**:11–16.
24. Centers for Disease Control. Pelvic inflammatory disease: Guidelines for prevention and management. *MMWR* 1991;**40**(No. RR-5):1–25.

3
Microbial Etiology of Pelvic Inflammatory Disease

RICHARD L. SWEET

Pelvic inflammatory disease (PID) is the most common major complication of sexually transmitted pathogens among young women and is associated with significant medical and economic consequences.[1] An estimated 1 million women are treated annually for PID in the United States[2,3]; in 1990 there were approximately 200,000 hospitalized cases of PID.[4] Washington and Katz[5] estimated that for 1990 annual costs associated with PID were $4.2 billion and projected that these costs would rise to approach $10 billion by the year 2000. Of increasing concern has been the recognition that significant adverse reproductive sequelae are associated with PID. One-fourth of women who experience an episode of acute PID subsequently develop one or more such long-term sequelae. The most common and most important of these is involuntary tubal factor infertility, which occurs in approximately 20%.[6,7] Ectopic pregnancies occur at a six- to tenfold increased rate following acute PID.[6] In addition, other important sequelae such as chronic pelvic pain, dyspareunia, pelvic adhesions, and inflammatory residua occur in 15% to 20% of cases. Such complications often lead to major surgical intervention, including total abdominal hysterectomy and bilateral salpingo-oophorectomy.

Prevention of these significant economic and medical consequences requires development of prevention and treatment plans that are based upon the microbial etiology of acute PID. However, attempts to determine the microbial etiology of acute PID have been compromised by several factors. First, the clinical diagnostic criteria for acute PID have neither been validated nor standardized in the literature. Second, the fallopian tubes, which are the crucial site of infection, are inaccessible for routine microbiological studies without use of invasive surgical procedures. Third, the majority of studies reported in the literature fail to attempt to identify all the potential pathogens that may be casually associated with acute PID, including *Neisseria gonorrhoeae*, *Chlamydia trachomatis*, anaerobic and facultative bacteria, genital tract mycoplasmas, and/or viral agents such as *Herpes simplex* and *Cytomegalovirus*.

Recently attention has been focused on "silent" or "atypical" PID, a term used to describe the condition in which women with documented tubal factor infertility provide no history of being diagnosed or treated for PID despite the presence of chronic inflammatory residua.[8] If this is actually an asymptomatic, silent infection or an atypical clinical presentation (e.g., abdominal pain, intermenstrual bleeding, mucopurulent endocervical discharge) that is unrecognized as PID remains unclear. Whether this entity is associated with the same microbial etiology as traditional clinically symptomatic PID remains to be elucidated. Initial studies suggest that *C. trachomatis* may be uniquely associated with these atypical or unrecognized infections.[9–16]

General Principles

The etiology of PID is generally acknowledged to be polymicrobic in nature.[17] While in the past, *N. gonorrhoeae* was held to be the primary etiological agent for PID, investigations over the past 20 years have demonstrated that a wide variety of microorganisms have been recovered from the upper genital tract of women with acute PID.[18–25] Among these organisms are *N. gonorrhoeae*, *C. trachomatis*, genital mycoplasmas, anaerobic and aerobic bacteria of the endogenous vaginal flora such as *Prevotella* (*Bacteroides*) species, *Peptostreptococci* sp, *Gardnerella vaginalis*, *Escherichia coli*, *Haemophilus influenzae*, and aerobic streptococci. Rice and Schachter[26] noted that the majority of proven cases of PID are associated with *N. gonorrhoeae* and/or *C. trachomatis*. Recently, Jossens et al.[27] confirmed this finding in a large series (*n* = 589) of hospitalized cases of acute PID in which an STD organism was present in 65% of cases with *N. gonorrhoeae* or *C. trachomatis* recovered from 324 (55%) and 129 (22%), respectively. In 30% of cases only anaerobic and/or facultative bacteria were isolated; in addition, anaerobic and/or facultative organisms were frequently (nearly 50%) recovered from the upper genital tract of patients with a sexually transmitted disease (STD) organism.[27] Similarly, Rice and Schachter[26] noted that 25% to 50% of PID cases do not have detectable chlamydial or gonococcal infection, but rather other anaerobic and facultative bacterial pathogens have been isolated from the upper genital tract. These authors reported that the non-STD organisms are similar to those associated with bacterial vaginosis.

The majority of PID cases occur as the result of intracanalicular spread of microorganisms from the endocervix and vagina to the endometrium and fallopian tubes.[28] In general, 10% to 17% of patients with cervical infection due to *N. gonorrhoeae* and *C. trachomatis* will develop PID.[29] In a few studies, up to 40% of women not treated for gonococcal or chlamydial cervicitis or who have been exposed to men with gonococcal or chlamydial urethritis develop clinical symptoms of PID.[30,31] With the use of endometrial biopsy to detect histological endometritis, higher percentages of subclinical ascending infection of the upper genital tract are present in women with gonococcal and/or chlamydial cervicitis.[28] Similarly, ascending infection of the endometrial cavity documented by the presence of histological endometritis occurs in women with bacterial vaginosis.[22,32,33]

In a recent review on PID, the Centers for Disease Control (CDC) listed four factors that may contribute to ascent of bacteria from the endocervix and vagina and/or be associated in the pathogenesis of PID.[28] These were: (1) Uterine instrumentation, especially insertion of intrauterine device (IUD), which facilitates upward spread of vaginal and cervical microorganisms; (2) Hormonal changes during menses and menstruation leads to cervical changes, resulting in loss of the mechanical barrier that helps prevent ascent of bacteria; (3) Retrograde menstruation favors ascent of bacteria from the endometrium to the fallopian tubes and peritoneal cavity; and (4) Individual microorganisms have potential virulence factors associated with development of PID.

For PID to develop, ascent of microorganisms from the lower genital tract through the internal cervical os, into the endometrial cavity, through the uterotubal junction and into the fallopian tubes must occur.[26,34] This intracannilicular spread of microorganisms is associated with a continuum of infection microbiologically and histologically that includes the cervix, endometrium, and fallopian tubes.[35] It is believed that the endocervical canal and the cervical mucus plug are the major barriers protecting the upper genital tract from microorganism present in the vagina and cervix.[26,36] Infection of the cervix with *C. trachomatis*, *N. gonorrhoeae* and/or other microorganisms could result in damage to the endocervical canal or breakdown of the cervical mucus plug thus leading to ascending infection.[26] While such a mechanism has been attributed to *N. gonorrhoeae* and *C. trachomatis*, Soper[22] recently proposed that bacterial vaginosis may facilitate ascent of STD and other aerobic bacteria through the cervical mucous barrier secondary to enzymatic degradation by proteolytic enzymes associated with the bacterial vaginosis (BV)-associated bacteria. An additional condition that might facilitate ascendance of microorganisms may be damage to the normal clearance mechanisms associated with ciliated epithelial cells in the endometrium and fallopian tube.[26]

The anatomy and physiology unique to females may combine to facilitate ascending infection with *N. gonorrhoeae*, *C. trachomatis*, and/or endogenous bacteria from the vagina.[26,36] As discussed in Chapter 2, young age is a major risk factor for PID. Cervical ectopy occurs more commonly in adolescents and results in a larger target area for attachment of *C. trachomatis*.[37,38] Rice and Schachter[26] suggested that other specific age-related changes in cervical mucus or other endocervical defense mechanisms may play a role in facilitating ascending infection. Hormonal changes associated with the normal menstrual cycle affect the potential for ascending infection via their effect on cervical mucus. At mid cycle when estrogen levels are high and progesterone low, cervical mucus may facilitate ascendance of infection while after ovulation high progesterone levels make the mucus thick and less penetrable to bacteria.[26,34] Moreover, with onset of menses the cervical mucus plug is lost and microorganisms from the vagina and cervix can ascend into the uterine cavity. Interestingly, the majority of symptomatic chlamydial and gonococcal PID cases have their onset during or just after the menses.[39,40] Last, retrograde menstruation has been proposed as a mechanism by which microorganisms from the endometrial cavity may be propelled into the fallopian tubes.[26]

Whether combination oral contraceptives alter the risk for PID is controversial.[26,32] Although women who use oral contraceptives may be at increased risk for cervical chlamydial infection,[26,37,38] most studies demonstrate that the incidence of PID as well as the clinical and laparoscopic severity of PID are reduced in patients using oral contraceptives.[26,41-45] *In vitro* studies have demonstrated that progesterone inhibits the growth of *N. gonorrhoeae*.[46-49] On the other hand, in animal models estrogen and progesterone facilitate the growth of *C. trachomatis* and ascendance of *C. trachomatis* into the upper genital tract.[26] As a result of these studies, concern has been raised that oral contraceptives may mask the signs and symptoms of ascending infection leading to an increase of subclinical cases that also are associated with tubal infertility and ectopic pregnancy.[26]

Primarily the host immune system protects against infection through rapid and efficient clearance of bacteria. However, the resultant inflammatory response may paradoxically lead to tissue damage or persistent infection.[26] For example, secretory IgA antigonococcal antibody inhibits attachment of *N. gonorrhoeae* to epithelial cells but interferes with phagocytosis of bacteria by *polymorphonuclearleukocytes* (PMNs). Similarly, oxygen metabolites (e.g., hypochlorite, superoxide anion, and hydrogen peroxide) produced when PMNs phagocytose bacteria, may cause tissue damage to the mucosal surface of the genital tract.[50] In addition, the cell-mediated immune response to bacteria, particularly *C. trachomatis*, may also result in a pathogenic mechanism leading to tissue damage in the fallopian tube.[26]

Neisseria Gonorrhoeae

In the United States, nontuberculous acute PID traditionally was separated into gonococcal and nongonococcal disease. This division was based solely on the recovery of *N. gonorrhoeae* from the endocervix of patients with acute PID. Studies utilizing endocervical cultures implicated the gonococcus as the causative agent in 33% to 81% of the cases of acute PID (Table 3.1).[17,29,51-60]

With *N. gonorrhoea*, the usual route of infection is thought to be a direct canalicular spread of the organism from the endocervix, along the endome-

TABLE 3.1. Frequency of endocervical GC in acute salpingitis patients.

	Total number of patients studied	Percent with gonorrhea
Holtz[53]	1,262	33
Jacobson and Weström[56]	563	40
Falk[54]	283	41
Hundley et al.[55]	80	41
Hedberg and Spetz[58]	216	44
Eschenbach et al.[61]	204	45
Sweet[29]	102	45
Lip and Burgoyne[57]	49	47
Cunningham et al.[52]	197	68
Thompson et al.[59]	30	80
Rendtorff[60]	111	81

trial surface to the tubal mucosa, leading to endosalpingitis. Approximately 10% to 17% of females who acquire endocervical gonorrhea will develop upper genital tract infection.[29,61]

The menstrual cycle may influence the environment of the lower genital tract and play a significant role in the breakdown of local host mechanisms that normally prevent the ascent of microorganisms from the endocervix. Two-thirds to three-fourths of the patients with gonococcal salpingitis present at the end of, or just after, the menstrual period.[40,61,62] Sweet et al.,[63] in a laparoscopy-based study, demonstrated an even more dramatic relationship between menses and gonococcal salpingitis. Although recovery of gonococcus from the cervix was most frequent within the first 7 days of the menstrual cycle, it was recovered from the cervix throughout the menstrual cycle. On the other hand, the gonococcus was isolated from the fallopian tubes only within the first 7 days after the onset of menses. Previously, it has been postulated that during the menstrual period, loss of the cervical mucous plug permitted microorganisms from the endocervix and vagina to gain access to the endometrial cavity. The bacteriostatic effect of cervical mucus is lowest at the onset of menses. Additionally, the endometrium, which may offer local protection against bacterial invasion, has been sloughed and menstrual blood from the endometrial cavity is an excellent culture medium. It has been postulated that gonococci either migrate into the fallopian tubes or are brought there by refluxed menstrual blood. Another possible mechanism, suggested by Toth et al.,[64] is the transport of gonococci via sperm attachment to the fallopian tubes. However, no data have been presented *in vivo* demonstrating that such a mechanism exists or that sperm can actually pick up bacteria from the vagina and/or cervix and bring them into the upper genital tract. Studies utilizing human fallopian tube organ cultures have shown that as gonococci reach the endosalpinx they become attached to mucosal epithelial cells, penetrate the epithelial cells, and cause cell destruction.[65–67] Within 2 to 7 days, ciliary motility is lost in fallopian tube organ cultures inoculated with *N. gonorrhoeae*. Gonococci selectively attach to and invade the nonciliated mucus-secreting cells of the fallopian tube epithelium.[66,67] In addition, Gregg et al. have demonstrated the production of an endotoxin (lipopolysaccharide) by the gonococcus that damages ciliated cells in human fallopian tube organ culture systems.[67] A second surface structural component of *N. gonorrhoeae*, peptidoglycan, has also been shown to damage the fallopian tube mucosa.[68]

Additional pathogenic mechanisms have been demonstrated for *N. gonorrhoeae*. Gonococci produce IgA proteases that breakdown secretory IgA, which binds to microorganisms and prevents their adherence to mucosal surfaces.[69] As a result, gonococcal adherence to mucosal cells is facilitated. *N. gonorrhoeae* also produce extracellular products such as phospholipase and peptidase, which are capable of producing cellular damage.[26] *N. gonorrhoeae* induces production of interferon-gamma, which in turn induces expression of major histocompatibility complex class II Ia antigens on epithelial cells. Expression of IA results in activation of the humoral and cell-mediated immune response that is directed against these epithelial cells.[26] Possibly this immune response is another mechanism by which *N. gonorrhoeae* destroys fallopian tube epithelial cells infected with the organism.[26,70] Grifo et al.[70] demonstrated that interferon-gamma was present in the serum in 65% of women with acute PID compared with none of healthy female controls.

Inherent properties of *N. gonorrhoeae* may also determine its ability to produce upper genital tract disease. It has been postulated that different strains of gonococci exist and that a particular strain(s) may be the virulent one for the development of salpingitis. This concept holds for disseminated gonorrhea in which the strain producing disseminated disease varies by microbiological susceptibility patterns and auxotypes from the organism, causing asymptomatic lower genital tract disease. Sweet and coworkers[71,72] studied virulence factors in paired fallopian tube-peritoneal cavity and endocervical isolates of *N. gonorrhoeae* obtained from patients with acute PID undergoing laparoscopy. Specifically, auxotypes (nutritional requirements), antimicrobial susceptibility, serum bactericidal activity, and colony phenotype were studied. Similar to the finding with disseminated gonorrhea, the gonococci recovered from women with PID had significantly different auxotypes and antimicrobial susceptibility patterns compared to those with uncomplicated anogenital disease. In contradistinction to the findings with disseminated gonorrhea, the gonococci causing acute PID were relatively more resistant to multiple antimicrobial agents, and the auxotype pattern most associated with acute PID was the prototrophic pattern (i.e., no extra amino acids required for growth), whereas the arginine hypoxanthine and uracil auxotype pattern was associated with uncomplicated lower genital tract gonorrhea. However, there was no difference among paired peritoneal cavity/cervical isolates of *N. gonorrhoeae* recovered from salpingitis patients relative to auxotypes and antimicrobial susceptibility patterns. The potential virulence factor that was significantly different in the paired fallopian tube endocervical gonorrhea specimens was colony phenotype.[71] Gonococci in the fallopian tube of women with acute salpingitis tended to be the transparent colony phenotype, whereas those present in the cervix of the same women tended to be opaque. In previous studies, women cultured during the menstrual cycle, except during the time of the menses, had a preponderance of opaque organisms isolated with a peak at the time of ovulation. The organisms usually recovered from the male urethra are heavily opaque, and the organisms recovered from women on oral contraceptives are opaque (women on oral contraceptives appear to be protected against the development of upper genital tract disease if they acquire gonorrhea).

Thus, epidemiologically and clinically, it appears that it is the transparent colony phenotypes that are the virulent form in the pathogenesis of acute salpingitis. To test this hypothesis, human fallopian tube and cervical organ culture explant systems have been used to evaluate endocervical and fallopian tube attachment. For the endocervix and fallopian tubes, the transparent colony phenotype of N. gonorrhoeae attaches more avidly than their opaque colony phenotype counterparts.[73] Possibly something in the cervical milieu, (hormones, pH, or an unidentified factor), may either select out the transparent colony phenotype or selectively drive the gonococci from opaque to transparent forms. In addition to colony phenotype (opaque or transparent), N. gonorrhoeae colony type are differentiated by the presence or absence of pili,[74,75] with the piliated strains appearing to be pathogenic.[74,75]

Chlamydia Trachomatis

C. trachomatis has received considerable attention as an etiological agent in acute PID over the past decade. Studies in Scandinavian countries were the first to demonstrate an important role for C. trachomatis in the etiology of acute PID[76–85] (Table 3.2). These studies reported the recovery of C. trachomatis from the cervix in 22% to 47% of women with acute PID. Of more interest, C. trachomatis was recovered from the fallopian tube(s) in 9% to 30% of women with visually confirmed acute PID[76,77,83] (Table 3.2). In addition, Scandinavian studies utilizing serological surveillance have demonstrated that C. trachomatis is associated with 23% to 62% of acute PID cases.[76,78–85]

Initial investigations in the United States failed to confirm the finding that chlamydia was a major causative agent in the etiology of acute PID. Eschenbach and coworkers[52] recovered C. trachomatis from the peritoneal cavity in only 1 of 54 cases, despite a 20% isolation rate of this organism from the cervix. Thompson et al.[59] showed that 10% of women with acute

TABLE 3.2. *Chlamydia trachomatis* in acute pelvic inflammatory disease.

Study	No. of patients	Isolation rate of *C. trachomatis*		Fourfold rise in serum antibodies (%)
		Endocervix (%)	Upper genital and peritoneal cavity (%)	
Eilard et al.[76]	22	6 (27)	2 (9)*	5 (23)
Mardh et al.[77]	53	19 (37)	6/20 (30)*	
Treharne et al.[78]	143			88 (62)[†]
Paavonen et al.[79]	106	27/26		19/72 (26)
Paavonen[80]	228	68 (30)		32/167 (19)
Mardh et al.[81]	60	23 (38)		24/60 (40)
Ripa et al.[82]	206	52/156 (33)		118 (57)[‡]
Gjonnaess et al.[83]	56	26 (46)	5/42 (12)*	26/52 (46)
Møller et al.[84]	166	37 (22)		34 (21)
Osser and Persson[85]	111	52 (47)		37/72 (51)
Eschenbach et al.[52]	100	20 (20)	1/54 (2)[§]	15/74 (20)
Sweet et al.[58]	37	2 (5)	0*	5/22 (23)
Thompson et al.[59]	30	3 (10)	3 (10)[‖]	
Sweet et al.[19]	71	10 (14)	17 (24)[¶]	
Wasserheit et al.[20]	22	10 (45)	8 (36)[¶]	
Kiviat et al.[88]	55	12 (22)	12 (22)[¶]	
Brunham et al.[25]	50	7 (14)	4 (8)[‖]	20 (40)
Landers et al.[123]	148	41 (28)	32 (22)[¶]	
Soper et al.[137]	84	13 (15)	1 (1)[‖]	
			6 (7)[¶]	
Kiviat et al.[88]	69		16 (23)	

*Fallopian tube.
[†]Chlamydial IgG ≥ 1:64; 23% had IgM ≥ 1:8.
[‡]Chlamydial IgG ≥ 1:64; fourfold rise in 28/80(35%).
[§]Culdocentesis.
[‖]Exudate from fallopian tube.
[¶]Fallopian tube and/or endometrial cavity.

PID had chlamydia isolated from the culdocentesis aspirates. In the first laparoscopy study performed in the United States, Sweet and coworkers[58] failed to recover *C. trachomatis* from the fallopian tube exudate in 37 patients. On the other hand, serological data from studies in the United States showed a fourfold rise in chlamydial antibodies in approximately 20% of acute cases.[52,58] Thus, until recently, most evidence in support of chlamydia as a major factor in acute salpingitis in the United States was indirect and derived from endocervical isolation and immunological studies. The contradictory results from Scandinavia and the United States were felt to be due to several factors. In Sweden, specimens for chlamydial cultures were obtained via biopsy or needle aspiration of the fallopian tube; in the United States, studies had utilized cultures from peritoneal fluid and/or tubal exudate. *C. trachomatis* is an intracellular organism, and, thus, fresh infected cells, such as obtained via biopsy, may be necessary to recover the organism. Second, the patient population studied may be different; the Swedish investigators studied women with a milder disease than usually was admitted to hospitals and studied in the United States. In fact, it has been suggested by Svensson and colleagues[82] that patients with milder PID are more likely to have *C. trachomatis* as the causative agent. These investigators noted that the women with *C. trachomatis* as the causative agent were more likely to be afebrile and have longer standing disease of milder type than women with gonococcal or nongonococcal, nonchlamydial disease. Paradoxically though, at laparoscopy, those women with *C. trachomatis* infection based on serological data had the most severe fallopian tube involvement and the highest estimated erythrocyte sedimentation rates (ESR).[86]

Recent studies have demonstrated a definite role for *C. trachomatis* as an etiological agent for acute PID in the United States and Canada. Bowie,[87] in a sexually transmitted disease clinic population in Vancouver, reported that women diagnosed to have acute PID had *C. trachomatis* recovered from their cervix significantly more often than women attending the clinic who did not have pelvic inflammatory disease. In this report, *C. trachomatis* was recovered from the cervix in 50% of women diagnosed as having acute PID, compared with 20% of women attending the STD clinic who did not have acute PID. More pertinent has been the direct evidence provided by Sweet and coworkers[19] utilizing specimens obtained from the upper genital tract (endometrial cavity and/or fallopian tubes) of hospitalized women with acute PID. These investigators recovered *C. trachomatis* from 17 (24%) of 71 of these patients. In an updated series of 380 patients with acute PID, *C. trachomatis* was recovered from the upper genital tract in 18%. Confirmation of a major role for *C. trachomatis* in the etiology of acute PID in the United States has been provided by Wasserheit and colleagues,[20] who reported that 14 (61%) of 23 women with salpingitis and/or plasma cell endometritis had *C. trachomatis* identified in the upper genital tract. Similarly, Kiviat et al.[88] and Landers et al.[89] recovered *C. trachomatis* from the upper genital tract in 22% and 22% of PID patients, respectively. Thus, clinicians must appreciate that current evidence strongly supports a putative role for *C. trachomatis* in acute salpingitis.

Recent information further suggests that chlamydia may play a possible role in infertility due to tubal obstruction and salpingitis.[9–16,90–92] These studies (see Table 3.3) have demonstrated in a wide variety of populations and geographic areas that women with tubal factor infertility are significantly more likely to have had previous systemic chlamydial infection than pregnant controls or nontubal factor infertility patients. A similar association with previous chlamydial infection and ectopic pregnancy also has been demonstrated recently[11,93–95] (Table 3.4). Thus, the two major sequelae of acute PID, tubal infertility and ectopic pregnancy, have been associated with prior chlamydial infection. Although suggestive for a direct etiological role in tubal infertility for *C. trachomatis*, these seroepidemiological studies do not prove causation.

TABLE 3.3. Studies demonstrating an association between *Chlamydia trachomatis* infection and infertility.

Study (yr)	Location	Study populations	Antichlamydial antibody (%)
Punnonen et al.[90] (1979)*	Finland	Infertile women with abnormal HSG	91
		Infertile women with normal HSG	51
Henry–Suchet et al.[91] (1980)†	Paris	Infertile women with tubal obstruction	26
		Infertile women without tubal obstruction	4
Jones et al.[9] (1982)*	Indianapolis	Infertile women with chlamydia antibody	75
		Infertile women without chlamydia antibody	28
Moore et al.[10] (1982)†	Seattle	Infertile women with tubal occlusions	75
		Infertile women without tubal occlusions	0
Cevenini et al.[12] (1982)*	Italy	Infertile women with salpingitis	90
		Infertile women without salpingitis	27
Gump et al.[11] (1983)*	Burlington	Infertile women with abnormal HSG	64
		Infertile women with normal HSG	28
Conway et al.[14] (1984)†	England	Tubal factor infertility	75
		Infertility—not tubal factor	31
Kane et al.[15] (1984)*	England	Infertile women with hydrosalpinx	41
		Infertility—not tubal factor	12
Brunham et al.[92] (1985)†	Winnipeg	Tubal factor infertility	72
		Infertility—not tubal factor	9
Sellors et al.[16] (1988)‡	Hamilton	Women undergoing tuboplasty	81
		Women with tubal ligation	37

* MIF ≥ 1:8. MIF = Microimmunofluorescence.
† MIF ≥ 1:32.
‡ EIA = Enzyme Immunoassay.
§ Percent with tubal obstruction.

Animal model studies have provided further evidence that supports the role of *C. trachomatis* in the etiology and pathogenesis of acute PID.[96–101] These have included use of the guinea pig inclusion conjunctivitis (GPIC) agent in the guinea pig, the mouse pneumonia biovar of *C. trachomatis* in the mouse, and human *C. trachomatis* in the Grivet monkey.[97,99,101]

It is generally held that chlamydial salpingitis, similar to the situation in gonococcal salpingitis, results from the intracanalicular spread of

TABLE 3.4. Relationship of previous chlamydial infection and ectopic pregnancy.

Author	Location	Study groups	Chlamydial antibody (%)
Gump et al.[11] (1983)*	Burlington	Ectopic pregnancy rate Infertility patients seropositive	32
		Ectopic preganancy rate Infertility patients seronegative	4
Svensson et al.[94] (1985)[†]	Sweden	Ectopic pregnancy	65
		Intrauterine pregnancy	21
		Male factor infertility	11
Brunham et al.[93] (1986)[†]	Winnipeg	Ectopic pregnancy	56
		Pregnant women	22
Hartford et al.[95†]	Los Angeles	Ectopic with disease in contralateral tube	50
		Ectopic with normal contralateral tube	0
Walters et al.[157] (1988)[†]	San Antonio	Ectopic pregnancy	66
		Intrauterine pregnancy	20
Chow et al.[158] (1990)[†]	Los Angeles/ San Francisco	Ectopic pregnancy Intrauterine pregnancy	71 39

* MIF ≥ 1:8.
[†] MIF ≥ 1:32.

C. trachomatis from the endocervix to the endometrium and hence to the fallopian tube.[16,54,102] Ripa et al.[97] have shown that *C. trachomatis* in a Grivet monkey model gains access to the fallopian tube mucosa as an ascending intracanalicular infection from the endocervix. Toth et al.[64] have reported that *C. trachomatis* attach to sperm and suggested that sperm may well be the vector that facilitates spread of microorganisms, including chlamydia, into the upper genital tract. However, actual attachment of *C. trachomatis* was not proven. Moreover, no study has demonstrated that sperm can carry *C. trachomatis* into the upper genital tract *in vivo*. Recently, an association between chlamydial salpingitis and menstruation, similar to that for *N. gonorrhoeae*, has been noted.[39] In this study, among the women who developed acute PID within 7 days from the onset of menses, 81% had chlamydial and/or gonococcal infection. In addition, 50% of chlamydial infection occurred within 7 days of the onset of menses. Thus, it appears that the pathogenesis of chlamydial salpingitis parallels that seen in gonococcal disease. No specific virulence factors that facilitate the development of acute PID have been identified for *C. trachomatis*.

Unlike the situation with most bacterial infections where tissue damage results from the direct effect of bacterial replication, the damage and scarring associated with *C. trachomatis* is the result of the host immune response to the infection.[103–107] Patton et al.,[103] in a monkey model, demonstrated that primary chlamydial infection is associated with a mild to moderate inflammation with an influx of polymorphonuclear cells. This is a self-limited infection that peaks by 2 weeks and resolves within 5 weeks.[103] On the other hand, repeated inoculations with *C. trachomatis* results in an infection and inflammation, characterized by mononuclear cells and formation of lymphoid follicles.[104] Rather than a self-limited infection with complete resolution, repeated infection in this monkey model produces extensive tubal scarring, distal tubal obstruction, and peritubal adhesions.[104] Such scarring of the fallopian tube subsequently leads to tubal infertility and/or ectopic pregnancy.[26]

Recent investigations have identified a *C. trachomatis* specific 57-KD protein that is responsible for this inflammatory response.[108,109] As noted by Møller et al.[108,110] the histopathology of the inflammatory response to this 57-KD protein is similar in human fallopian tube tissue to that seen in blinding trachoma and genital tract models of infertility. This 57-KD protein has been identified as a heat shock protein[26] and has been shown to induce a hypersensitivity response in the conjunctiva of ocular immune guinea pigs.[108] Wager et al. have demonstrated that women with PID or ectopic pregnancy have antibodies against this protein.[111] Similarly, Brunham and coworkers[112] reported that patients with tubal factor infertility have antibodies directed at the 57-KD antigen and Witkin et al.[113] reported that induction of a cell-mediated immune response to the chlamydial 57-KD heat shock protein is a common feature of upper genital tract infection. Recently Patton et al.[114] demonstrated that *C. trachomatis* infection in monkeys induced delayed hypersensitivity that is mediated by *C. trachomatis* heat shock protein (hsp 60). Thus, the pathogenesis of acute PID and trachoma due to infection with *C. trachomatis* are similar.[26,113,115]

Anaerobic and Facultative Bacteria

It has become evident that the presence of pathogenic microorganisms in the endocervix is not absolute proof that such microorganisms are causally associated with upper genital tract infections such as salpingitis. Investigations utilizing transvaginal culdocentesis and laparoscopy to obtain culture specimens from the peritoneal fluid or fallopian tube exudate have demonstrated a poor correlation between the cervical and intra-abdominal cultures. Despite isolation from the endocervix of patients with acute salpingitis, *N. gonorrhoeae* was recovered from only 6% to 70% of the peritoneal and/or tubal cultures.[23,52,57,116-120] Investigations in the late 1970s utilizing culdocentesis and appropriate anaerobic culture techniques led to the isolation of a variety of aerobic and anaerobic bacteria from the peritoneal fluid of patients with acute PID.[17,23,52,57-59,63,117,119] The most frequent organisms recovered in these studies were *N. gonorrhoeae* and anaerobic bacteria, including *Peptostreptococcus*, and *Bacteroides* (*Prevotella*) species. A characteristic pattern evolved from these studies (Table 3.5). Although there was a high prevalence of *N. gonorrhoeae* in the cervix of these patients, less than one-fourth of the cases had *N. gonorrhoeae* as the only organism recovered from an intra-abdominal site. An additional one-fourth of the patients had a mixture of *N. gonorrhoeae* plus mixed anaerobic and aerobic bacteria (predominantly anaerobes). The final 50% of the patients did not have *N. gonorrhoeae*, but only a mixture of anaerobic and aerobic bacteria were recovered from the abdominal cavity. These culdocentesis studies demonstrated that the etiology of acute PID is polymicrobic in nature and brought into question the exact role of *N. gonorrhoeae* in the pathogenesis of acute pelvic inflammatory disease. Cunningham et al.,[52] Chow et al.,[117] and Monif et al.[119] postulated that the gonococcus initiates the inflammatory process and produces tissue damage and changes in the local environment, which in turn allow access to the upper genital tract for anaerobic and aerobic organisms from the vaginal and cervical flora. On the other hand, McCormack et al.,[62] Eschenbach,[51] and Sweet et al.[23] have suggested that not all pelvic inflammatory disease follows gonococcal infection and that, in fact, acute pelvic inflammatory disease initially has a polymicrobial etiology. At the other extreme, Soper et al.[22] have suggested that BV, an overgrowth of anaerobic and aerobic flora of the vagina, may predispose or facilitate the ascent of *N. gonorrhoeae* into the upper genital tract.

It is uncertain that microorganisms obtained from cul-de-sac fluid, aspirated transvaginally, are truly representative of the microorganisms present in the fallopian tube. A study by Sweet et al.[63] demonstrated a discrepancy between culdocentesis and fallopian tube isolates from females with acute PID. Culdocentesis specimens yielded greater numbers of bacteria common to the vaginal flora than did the fallopian tube isolates. In a subsequent study in which 10 patients had cultures from the fallopian tube and the cul-de-sac obtained via laparoscopy, and the cul-de-sac obtained via transvaginal culdocentesis, close agreement was noted between fallopian

TABLE 3.5. Isolation of *N. gonorrhoeae*, anaerobes, and aerobes from culdocentesis aspirates in acute pelvic inflammatory disease.

Study	No. of patients	Endocervical *N. gonorrhoeae* (%)	Culdocentesis		
			N. gonorrhoeae only (%)	*N. gonorrhoeae* plus anaerobes and aerobes (%)	Anaerobes and aerobes only (%)
Cunningham et al.[52]	104	56 (54)	12 (22)	18 (32)	26 (46)
Thompson et al.[59]	30	24 (80)	5 (21)	5 (21)	14 (58)
Eschenbach et al.[17]	54	21 (39)	6 (28)	1 (5)	5 (24)
Monif et al.[119]	17	16 (94)	5 (31)	5 (31)	6 (38)
Sweet et al.[63]	26	13 (50)	4 (31)	4 (31)	4 (31)
Chow et al.[117]	20	13 (65)		1 (5)	18 (95)
Total	251	143 (57)	32 (23)	34 (24)	73 (52)

TABLE 3.6. Distribution of microorganisms isolated from women with acute pelvic inflammatory disease at San Francisco General Hospital (based on data from reference 23).

Microorganisms	Fallopian tube (N = 35)		Culdocentesis (N = 35)		Endocervix (N = 35)	
	No.	%	No.	%	No.	%
N. gonorrhoeae	8	23	11	31	19	49
N. gonorrhoeae only	6	17	3	8.5		
N. gonorrhoeae in combination with other bacteria	2	6	8	23		
Aerobic bacteria only	1	3	1	3		
Anaerobic bacteria	10	29	20	57		
Anaerobes only	3	8.5	5	14		
Mixed anaerobes/ aerobes	7	20	15	43		
M. hominis	0		1	3	28	80
U. urealyticum	3	8.5	6	17	21	60
C. trachomatis	0		0		2	5
No growth	13	37	9	26		

tube exudate and the cul-de-sac aspirate via laparoscopy, but there was poor correlation with the culdocentesis results, suggesting that contamination may occur during transvaginal culdocentesis.[23] Soper et al.[121] have confirmed this finding that use of culdocentesis to obtain a microbiological specimen from the peritoneal cavity is fraught with the problem of contamination by the vaginal flora.

The optimum microbiological information for elucidating the etiology of acute PID would be obtained using specimens obtained directly from the site of infection—the fallopian tubes and/or endometrial cavity. In 1980, Sweet and coworkers[23] reported their results from the first laparoscopy study of PID performed in the United States with cultures obtained directly from the fallopian tube. These results are presented in Table 3.6. While nearly 50% of the patients had N. gonorrhoeae recovered from the endocervix, the gonococcus was isolated from the fallopian tube in only 8 of 35 patients (23%). Anaerobic bacteria were the most frequent fallopian tube isolates from these females with acute salpingitis. Anaerobes were recovered in 10 cases (29%); Peptostreptococcus species were the most prevalent anaerobes. Since this initial report, we have described the microbiological results of cultures obtained from the upper genital tract (endometrial aspirates and/or fallopian tube specimens) of an additional 380 hospitalized women with acute PID (Table 3.7).[1,19,122,123] N. gonorrhoeae and C. trachomatis were recovered from 45% and 18%, respectively. However, nongonococcal (NG), nonchlamydial (NC) bacteria were the most frequently recovered organisms and were present in 70% of cases. Again, anaerobic bacteria were the predominant isolates. The NG, NC

TABLE 3.7. Microbiologic results from hospitalized patients with acute pelvic inflammatory disease at San Francisco General Hospital

Organism	No. of patients positive/No. of patients cultured	% Positive
N. gonorrhoeae	172/380	45
C. trachomatis	68/380	18
M. hominis	34/87	39
U. urealyticum	13/87	15
Nongonococcal, nonchlamydial bacteria	267/380*	70

*Primary plate isolates.

organisms identified are noted in Table 3.8. The most common included *Bacteroides* (*Prevotella*) species, *Bacteroides* (*Prevotella*) *bivius*, *Bacteroides* (*Prevotella*) *disiens*, *Peptostreptococcus* sp., *Gardnerella vaginalis*, group B streptococcus, and *Escherichia coli*.

Frequent isolation of anaerobic and facultative (aerobic) bacteria from the upper genital tract of women with acute PID has been confirmed by recent studies in Scandinavia and the United States. Heinonnen et al.[24] reported that although *C. trachomatis* was the most common individual organism recovered from the fallopian tubes and endometria of patients with acute PID, NG NC bacteria were the most commonly recovered group of microorganisms (Table 3.9). Similar findings from Scandinavia have been reported by Paavonen and coworkers.[124] In the United States, Wasserheit

TABLE 3.8. Nongoncococcal, nonchlamydial bacteria recovered from the upper genital tract of patients with acute salpingitis at San Francisco General Hospital ($N = 188$).

Organism	No. of patients
Bacteroides species	88
B. bivius	72
B. disiens	25
Other *Bacteroides*	99
Peptostreptococcus asaccharolyticus	93
Peptostreptococcus anaerobius	71
G. vaginalis	121
E. coli	25
Nonhemolytic streptococci	49
Group B streptococci	29
α-hemolytic streptococci	45
Coagulase-negative staphylococci	72

and colleagues[20] demonstrated that anaerobic and/or aerobic bacteria were recovered from the upper genital tract in 44% of patients with acute PID. Brunham et al.[125] in a Canadian study, and Soper et al.[22] in a United States study, reported a lower recovery of mixed anaerobic and facultative bacteria from the fallopian tubes with rates of 20% and 13%, respectively. However, Soper et al.[22] noted that anaerobic and facultative organisms were isolated from the endometrial cavity in 31.4% of their laparoscope confirmed cases of PID. In addition, Paavonen et al.[126] reported that significant enterobacterial common antigen and *B. fragilis* antibody titers were present in one-third of patients with PID, supporting the concept that anaerobes and aerobes are involved in the etiology of PID.

These investigations demonstrating isolation of a variety of bacteria other than *N. gonorrhoeae* from several different intra-abdominal sites, most notably the fallopian tubes, provide support for the concept of the polymicrobial etiology of acute PID. This has led to a reevaluation of the role of the gonococcus in the pathogenesis of acute salpingitis. It was a common belief that as the duration of symptoms increased, the microflora of the fallopian tube changed from *N. gonorrhoeae* (the initiator of disease and tubal destruction) to the secondary invaders, such as the facultative and anaerobic bacterial flora from the lower genital tract. This concept was initially proposed in 1921 by Curtis, who found *N. gonorrhoeae* only in cases that showed microscopic evidence of active inflammation at operation, but not in patients that had been afebrile for 14 days.[127] Curtis concluded that gonococci survived only a short time in the fallopian tube. Similarly Lip and Burgoyne reported that the isolation of *N. gonorrhoeae* was dependent on the stage of infection.[57] They were unable to isolate the gonococcus if symptoms had been present for 7 days or more. Therefore, it is possible that acute PID patients admitted to the hospital after several days of symptoms have already passed through an initial stage, in which *N. gonorrhoeae* participates as a primary pathogen, after which they progressed to a mixed

TABLE 3.9. Recovery of microorganisms from the upper genital tract of patients with acute PID.

Study	No. of patients	*Chlamydia trachomatis* No. (%)	*Neisseria gonorrhoeae* No. (%)	Anaerobic and aerobic bacteria No. (%)
Sweet[19,23,63,122]	380	68 (18)	172 (45)	267 (70)
Wasserheit[20]	23	11 (44)	8 (35)	11 (44)
Heinonnen[24]	25	10 (40)	4 (16)	17 (68)
Paavonen[21]	35	12 (34)	4 (11)	24 (69)
Brunham[25]	50	21 (42)	8 (16)	10 (20)
Soper[22]	84*	1 (1.2)	32 (38)	12 (13)
	51†	6 (7.4)	49 (98)	16 (32)

*Fallopian tube/cul-de-sac.
†Endometrial cavity.

aerobic/anaerobic infection involving secondary invading pathogens from the cervix and vagina. Based upon fallopian tube specimens, Sweet et al.[120] demonstrated that 70% of patients presenting within the initial 24 h from the onset of symptoms had *N. gonorrhoeae* present. Anaerobic bacteria were present in the fallopian tubes within the initial 24 h of symptoms as well. If symptoms had been present for greater than 24 h, there appeared to be a shift in the bacteria isolated from the fallopian tube: anaerobic bacteria and *Ureaplasma urealyticum* became predominant. If symptoms had been present for greater than 48 h, we could recover the gonococcus from only 19% of patients ($p < 0.001$). Thus, direct cultures from the fallopian tube failed to confirm the initial concept that anaerobes would be secondary invaders. In patients presenting with less than 24 h of symptomatology, mixtures of anaerobic and aerobic bacteria were recovered in 37% of the patients. This ability to recover anaerobes from the fallopian tube persisted during subsequent duration of disease. In a small number of patients (three), anaerobic bacteria were the most common fallopian tube isolates within the first 24 h of onset of symptoms: neither *N. gonorrhoeae* nor *C. trachomatis* were isolated from the tubes or cervix of these patients. Therefore, it appears that NG, NC bacteria from the cervix and vagina may also be present early in the disease process. If the gonococcus were the initiator, we would expect an inverse relationship between the frequency of isolation of *N. gonorrhoeae* and anaerobic bacteria; this relationship does not seem to exist. Soper and coworkers[22] recently reported in 84 patients with laparoscopy confirmed salpingitis that no correlation existed between the duration of symptoms and the presence of *N. gonorrhoeae* or upper genital tract anaerobes. Eschenbach and Holmes[128] and Monif[129] also were not able to demonstrate a direct correlation between duration of symptoms and microbial etiology.

Many of the NG, NC microorganisms recovered from the upper genital tract of patients with acute PID also have been implicated in BV (formerly nonspecific vaginitis), a complex synergistic vaginal infection associated with *G. vaginalis*, *Prevotella* (*Bacteroides*) species (especially *P. bivius*, *P. disiens*, and *P. capillosus*), *Peptostreptococcus* sp., the mobile curved anaerobic rod *Mobiluncus* sp., alpha-hemolytic streptococci, and *M. hominis*.[130-134] Eschenbach initially postulated that BV might be an antecedent precursor in the lower genital tract for the development of NG, NC PID.[51] There have been several investigations that have demonstrated an association between BV and PID.[33,135-137] Paavonen and coworkers[135] reported that 9 (29%) of 31 women with laparoscope confirmed acute PID had BV compared with 0 of 14 controls. Moreover, all 9 of these women had histological endometritis present on endometrial biopsy. Subsequently, Eschenbach et al.[136] demonstrated that women with BV were significantly more likely to have adnexal tenderness (4% vs. 0.3%), uterine tenderness (4% vs. 1%), cervical motion tenderness (3% vs. 0.6%) and a diagnosis of PID (3% vs. 0%) than control women without BV. These authors controlled for age, race, parity, education, smoking, sexual behavior, and coinfection. Hillier and colleagues[33] reported that the BV-associated micro-organisms (*Prevotella*, Peptostreptococcus, and *M. hominis*) were associated with histological endometritis in confirmed cases of PID. Even after controlling for chlamydial and gonococcal infection, the recovery of BV-associated bacteria from the endometrial cavity was independently associated with histological endometritis.[33] Recently, Soper et al.[137] noted in women with laparoscopy confirmed PID that BV was present in 61.8%. In addition, all the anaerobes recovered from the upper genital tract in their study were the BV-associated microorganisms.[137] Interestingly, a higher incidence of BV has been noted in women wearing IUDs than among noncontraceptors or women using other contraceptive methods.[138,139] Such an association may play a role in the pathogenesis of nongonococcal nonchlamydial PID.

Little of the pathogenesis in NG, NC salpingitis has been elucidated. Recent reports have shown that PID is a polymicrobial infection, and the organisms implicated include aerobic and anaerobic bacteria. The cervix and vagina of healthy women have been shown to contain a multitude of aerobic and anaerobic bacteria.[140] How these organisms gain access to the upper genital tract is not known. As postulated for *N. gonorrhoeae*, they may reach the fallopian tube in menstrual blood reflux or attach to sperm. Eschenbach[61] has suggested that there may be a critical number of organisms needed to overwhelm local host defense mechanisms in the cervix, thereby allowing an infection to ascend to the upper genital tract. There appears to be a continuum from the entity of BV, which is associated with significantly increased and high colony counts of anaerobic bacteria and *Gardnerella vaginalis* and NG, NC salpingitis. Such a scenario is reinforced by the microbiology results presented by Sweet and coworkers.[19] These investigators recovered *G. vaginalis* from the upper genital tract in 30 (40%) of 74 hospitalized women with acute salpingitis. This organism was nearly always found in association with anaerobic bacteria, particularly *Prevotella* (*Bacteroides*) species, *P. bivius*, and anaerobic cocci. A hypothesis that requires confirmation is that the synergistic infection with anaerobes and *G. vaginalis* may be a third (in addition to *N. gonorrhoeae* and *C. trachomatis*) instance in which a lower genital tract infection ascends into the upper genital tract and produces acute salpingitis. Even if such a hypothesis is not confirmed, it is apparent that NG, NC bacteria are involved in the etiology and pathogenesis of acute salpingitis.[19,52,58] Moreover, as demonstrated by the laparoscopy study of Sweet and coworkers,[120] the NG, NC organisms can cause acute salpingitis without antecedent infection with *N. gonorrhoeae* and/or *C. trachomatis*. Although not identified yet, some alteration in the normal cervical defense mechanism must occur that allows microorganisms from the cervix and vagina to gain access to the upper genital tract. Perhaps cervical infection with *N. gonorrhoeae* and/or *C. trachomatis* produces such a change.

The pathogenic mechanism of IUD-associated salpingitis is different from that seen with the gonococcus or chlamydia. When the IUD was reintroduced into clinical practice in 1959, it was postulated that infection would occur only at the time of insertion, with a break in sterile technique, or with the introduction of pathogenic bacteria. More recently, it has become apparent that the device alters the host defense mechanisms within the uterine cavity. There are a variety of ways in which an IUD can interfere with normal host defense mechanisms. These include: (1) breakdown of the mucosal surface in the endometrial cavity; (2) foreign body interference with the ability of polymorphic neutrophils (PMNs) to phagocytose bacteria; (3) development of a biofilm that protects bacteria from host defenses; (4) decreased concentration of bacteria required to produce infection; and (5) presence of minerals that can interfere with some components of the host defenses. In addition, recent studies have shown that the IUD string facilitates upward spread of bacteria, which allows organisms to ascend to the lower uterine segment.[141,142] In these studies the lower uterine segment has become colonized in patients using IUDs with strings, whereas it has not become colonized in those using IUDs without strings. Intrauterine device strings of multifilament nature have a greater propensity for attachment of bacteria and promotion of bacterial movement into the endometrial cavity.[142] This combination of the string facilitating ascension of bacteria from the lower genital tract and the presence of a foreign body interfering with local host defense mechanisms sets the stage in the uterine cavity for the development of endometritis and subsequent progressive endometritis, leading to salpingitis. These patients usually present with intermenstrual bleeding and crampy abdominal pain. Histologically, there are submucosal microabscesses beneath the area of the IUD placement.[143] Ober et al.[144] demonstrated that IUD wearers with symptoms of bleeding and crampy abdominal pain were significantly more likely to have histological endometritis than asymptomatic IUD users. Once an endometritis is established, the pathogenesis of infection is similar to that seen with non-IUD-associated acute PID. While previously it was believed that IUD infections were similar to postabortion or postpartum infections where bacteria ascend via lymphatics in the parametrial tissue and broad ligament to reach the tube and adnexa producing a perisalpingitis, it now is felt that direct spread of microorganisms from the infected or colonized uterine cavity to the fallopian tubes is the major pathogenic mechanism. It has been suggested that women with acute salpingitis in association with the IUD are at increased risk for the development of adnexal abscesses.[143] In addition, it was felt that these IUD infections tend to be unilateral compared with other types of PID, which tend to be bilateral. Landers and Sweet[145] reported that 70% of their series of 232 tuboovarian abscesses were unilateral; this was true for IUD and non-IUD users. Thus, it appears there is not an association between IUD use and unilateral adnexal infection.

One pelvic infection that is unique to IUD use is that due to *Actinomyces israeli*. This organism is associated with severe infection, extensive inflammatory response, abscess formation and fistula formation. Women using IUDs are at increased risk to have colonization (documented by Pap smear) with *A. israeli* in the lower genital tract.

Genital Tract Mycoplasmas

The genital tract mycoplasmas, *M. hominis*, *U. urealyticum*, and *M. genitalium* also have been suggested as potential pathogens in the etiology of acute salpingitis.[146-149] However, their role remains controversial. Although *M. hominis* and *U. urealyticum* have been frequently recovered from the lower genital tract of women with PID, no difference exists between the rates of isolation from the cervices of these patients and in sexually active control patients.[52,146] Moreover, the genital tract mycoplasmas have been recovered infrequently (2% to 10%) from the peritoneal cavity and/or fallopian tubes of patients with salpingitis.[52,58,147] Speculation as to a potential role for genital mycoplasmas in the etiology of PID has focused predominantly on *M. hominis*. Mardh and Weström[147] reported a cervical isolation rate for *M. hominis* of 52%; Eschenbach et al.[17] recovered *M. hominis* from the vagina and/or cervix in 145 (72%) of 204 women with acute PID and Møller et al.[148] recovered *M. hominis* from 91 (55%) of 166 PID cases. Serological studies have also suggested a role for *M. hominis* in the etiology of acute PID.[52,146-149] Antibodies to *M. hominis* were present in one-fourth to one-half of women with acute PID in these investigations. In addition to the low recovery rate from the fallopian tube, *in vitro* studies with fallopian tube explant systems have suggested that mycoplasmas may be commensals rather than pathogens in acute PID. Taylor–Robinson and Carney[150] demonstrated that despite proliferation of *M. hominis*, there was no apparent tubal damage produced. This is in contradistinction to the circumstance when *N. gonorrhoeae* is placed in a similar system and extensive epithelial damages occurs and the tubal epithelium is completely destroyed within 7 days. More recently, Hare and Barnes[151] have noted that the use of *Bacteroides fragilis* in the tubal explant system resulted in tubal destruction and epithelial destruction within 72–96 h. However, it is important to recognize that the *in vitro* fallopian tube explant system precludes the immune response and host defense mechanisms, which may be important in the pathogenesis of acute salpingitis.[152] Møller and coworkers,[153] working with a Grivet monkey model, noted that *M. hominis* results in a parametritis rather than an acute salpingitis, and this could possibly explain the failure to recover mycoplasmas except in a few cases from the fallopian tubes. Using scanning electron microscopy, Mardh et al.[154] showed that *M. hominis* induced pathological swelling in fallopian tube cilia in organ culture systems. Although results obtained with serological studies and cervical isolated approaches are suggestive, the role of the genital tract mycoplasmas in the etiology of acute PID remains unclear. Perhaps the mycoplasmas participate in acute PID as the result of their association with BV.

Viruses

The etiological role of viruses in acute PID has not been extensively studied. In particular, a potential role has been suggested for the viral agents—herpes simplex virus (HSV) II and cytomegalovirus (CMV). Laparoscopy studies in the United States by Sweet et al.[23] and Wasserheit et al.[20] failed to demonstrate the presence of HSV in the cervices or fallopian tubes of patients with acute PID. However, investigators in Finland reported on the recovery of HSV in several patients from the cervix and/or the upper genital tract of women with laparoscopy confirmed acute PID.[155,156] Wasserheit et al.[20] noted that CMV was recovered from the cervices in 6 (28%) of 22 women with acute PID. Moreover, they reported that CMV was associated with chlamydia cervicitis and postulated that chlamydial infection might reactivate latent CMV. While interesting, these findings require confirmation, and the role of viral agents in acute PID awaits further investigation.

Summary

PID is now recognized to be a polymicrobial infection. The sexually transmitted organisms *N. gonorrhoeae* and/or *C. trachomatis* are involved in the majority of cases. Anaerobic and facultative bacteria from the normal flora of the vagina and cervix are also commonly present in the upper genital tract of women with acute PID. These organisms appear to be associated with BV. In roughly one-third of PID cases only the anaerobic and facultative bacteria are involved. In addition, these organisms occur in nearly 50% of STD-associated PID cases as well. The role of genital mycoplasmas in the etiology of PID remains uncertain. As a result of understanding the microbial etiology of PID, appropriate antimicrobial therapy can be instituted. In general, this requires coverage for *N. gonorrhoeae*, *C. trachomatis*, and mixed anaerobic and aerobic bacteria.

References

1. Sweet RL. Pelvic inflammatory disease and infertility in women. *Infect Dis Clin North Am* 1987;**1**:199–215.
2. Curran JW. Economic consequences of pelvic inflammatory disease in the United States. *Am J Obstet Gynecol* 1980;**138**:848.

3. Jones OG, Saida AA, St. John RK. Frequency and distribution of salpingitis and pelvic inflammatory disease in short stay in hospitals in the United States. *Am J Obstet Gynecol* 1980;**138**:905.

4. Rolfs RT, Galaid E, Zaidi AA. Epidemiology of pelvic inflammatory disease: Trends in hospitalizations and office visits, 1979–1988, in *Joint Meeting of the Centers for Disease Control and National Institutes of Health about Pelvic Inflammatory Disease Prevention, Management and Research in the 1990s*. Bethesda, MD, September 4–5, 1990.

5. Washington AE, Katz P. Cost of and payment source for pelvic inflammatory diasese: Trends and projections, 1983 through 2000. *JAMA* 1991;**266**: 2565–2569.

6. Weström L. Incidence, prevalence, and trends of acute pelvic inflammatory disease and its consequences in industrialized countries. *Am J Obstet Gynecol* 1980;**138**:880.

7. Weström L. Effect of acute pelvic inflammatory disease on fertility. *Am J Obstet Gynecol* 1975;**122**:876.

8. Wølner-Hanssen P, Kiviat NB, Holmes KK. Atypical pain inflammatory disease: Subacute, chronic, or subclinical upper genital tract infection in women, in Holmes KK, Mardh P-A, Sparling PF, Wiesner PJ, Cates W Jr., Lemon SM, Stamm WE (eds): *Sexually Transmitted Disease*. New York, McGraw-Hill, 1990, pp 615–620.

9. Jones RB, Ardery BR, Hui SL, Cleary RE. Correlation between serum antichlamydial antibodies and tubal factor as a cause of infertility. *Fertil Steril* 1982;**38**:553.

10. Moore DE, Foy HM, Dalin JR, et al. Increased frequency of serum antibodies to *Chlamydia trachomatis* in infertility due to tubal disease. *Lancet* 1982;**2**:574.

11. Gump DW, Gibson M, Ashikaga T. Evidence of prior pelvic inflammatory disease and its relationship to *C. trachomatis* antibody and intrauterine contraceptive device use in infertile women. *Am J Obstet Gynecol* 1983;**146**:153.

12. Cevanini R, Possati G, LaPlaca M. *Chlamydia trachomatis* infection in infertile women, in Mardh P-A, Holmes KK, Oriel JD, Piot P, Schachter J (eds): *Chlamydial Infections*. Amsterdam, Elsevier Biomedical Press, 1982, pp 182–192.

13. Gibson M, Gump D, Ashikaga T, Hall B. Patterns of adnexal inflammatory damage: Chlamydia, the intrauterine device, and history of pelvic inflammatory disease. *Fertil Steril* 1984;**41**:47–51.

14. Conway D, Caul EO, Hall MR. Chlamydial serology in fertile and infertile women. *Lancet* 1984;**1**:191.

15. Kane JL, Woodland RM, Forsey T, et al. Evidence of chlamydial infection in infertile women with and without fallopian tube obstruction. *Fertil Steril* 1984;**42**:6.

16. Sellors JW, Mahoney J, Chernesky M, et al. *Chlamydia trachomatis* in fertile and infertile Canadian women, in *Chlamydia Infections, Sixth International Symposium Proceedings June 1986*. England, Cambridge University Press, 1986, p. 233.

17. Eschenbach DA, Buchanan T, Pollock HM, et al. Polymicrobial etiology of acute pelvic inflammatory disease. *N Engl J Med* 1975;**293**:166.

18. Mardh P-A, Lind I, Svensson L, et al. Antibodies to *Chlamydia trachomatis*, *Mycoplasma hominis* and *Neisseria gonorrhoeae* in serum from patients with acute salpingitis. *Br J Vener Dis* 1981;**57**:125–129.

19. Sweet RL, Schachter J, Robbie MO. Failure of beta-lactam antibiotics to eradicate *Chlamydia trachomatis* in the endometrium despite apparent clinical cure of acute salpingitis. *JAMA* 1983;**250**:2641–2645.

20. Wasserheit JN, Bell TA, Kiviat NB, et al. Microbiol causes of proven pelvic inflammatory disease and efficacy of clindamycin and tobramycin. *Ann Int Med* 1986;**104**:187–193.

21. Paavonen J, Teisala K, Heinonnen PK, et al. Microbiological and histopathological findings in acute pelvic inflammatory disease. *Brit J Obstet Gynecol* 1987;**94**:454–460.

22. Soper DE, Brockwell NJ, Dalton HP, Johnson D. Observations concerning the microbial etiology of acute salpingitis. *Am J Obstet Gynecol* 1994;**170**:1008–1017.

23. Sweet RL, Draper DL, Schachter J, et al. Microbiology and pathogenesis of acute salpingitis as determined by laparoscopy: What is the appropriate site to sample? *Am J Obstet Gynecol* 1980;**138**:985.

24. Heinonnen PK, Teisala K, Punnonen R, et al. Anatomic sites of upper genital tract infection. *Obstet Gynecol* 1985;**66**:384–390.

25. Brunham RC, Binns B, Guijon F, et al. Etiology and outcome of acute pelvic inflammatory disease. *J Infect Dis* 1988;**158**:510–517.

26. Rice PA, Schachter J. Pathogenesis of pelvic inflammatory disease. *JAMA* 1991;**266**:2587–2593.

27. Jossens MOR, Schachter J, Sweet RL. Risk factors associated with pelvic inflammatory disease of differing microbial etiologies. *Obstet Gynecol* 1994;**83**:989–997.

28. Centers for Disease Control. Pelvic inflammatory disease: Guidelines for prevention and management. *MMWR* 1991;**40**:1–25.

29. Sweet RL. Diagnosis and treatment of acute salpingitis. *J Reprod Med* 1977;**19**:21.

30. Platt R, Rich PA, McCormack WM. Risk of acquiring gonorrhea and prevalence of abnormal adnexal findings among women recently exposed to gonorrhea. *JAMA* 1983;**250**:3205–3209.

31. Stamm WE, Guinan ME, Johnson C, et al. Effect of treatment regimens for *Neisseria gonorrhoeae* on simultaneous infection with *Chlamydia trachomatis*. *N Engl J Med* 1984;**310**:545–549.

32. Washington AE, Goves S, Schachter J, Sweet RL. Oral contraceptives, *Chlamydia trachomatis* infection and pelvic inflammatory disease. *JAMA* 1985;**124**:2246–2250.

33. Hillier SL, Kiviat NB, Critchlow C, et al. Bacterial vaginosis-associated bacteria as etiologic agents of pelvic inflammatory disease (Abstract), in *Proceedings of the annual meeting Infectious Disease Society of Obstetrics and Gynecology*, San Diego, CA, August 6, 1992.

34. Rice PA, Weström LV. Pathogenesis and inflammatory response in pelvic inflammatory disease, in Berger GS, Westrom LV (eds): *Pelvic Inflammatory Disease*. New York, Raven Press, 1992, pp 35–47.

35. Weström L, Mardh P-A. Acute pelvic inflammatory disease, in Holmes KK, Mardh P-A, Sparling PF, Wiesner PJ (eds): *Sexually Transmitted Diseases*. New York, McGraw-Hill, 1990, pp 593–613.

36. Odeblad E. The functional structure of human cervical mucus. *Acta Obstet Gynecol* Scand 1968;**47**(suppl 1):57–59.

37. Svensson L, Weström L, Mardh P-A. *Chlamydia trachomatis* in women attending a gynecological outpatient clinic with lower genital tract infection. *Br J Vener Dis* 1981;**57**:259–262.
38. Harrison HR, Phil D, Costi M, et al. Cervical *Chlamydia trachomatis* infection in university women: Relationship to history of contraception, ectopy and cervicitis.
39. Fullilove RE, Fullilove MT, Bower BP, Gross SA. Risk of sexually transmitted diseases among black adolescent crack users in Oakland and San Francisco, CA. *JAMA* 1990;**263**:851–855.
40. Nolan GJ, Osborne N. Gonococcal infection in the female. *Obstet Gynecol* 1973;**42**:156.
41. Washington AE, Aral SO, Wølner-Hanssen P, Grimes DA, Holmes KK. Assessing risk for pelvic inflammatory disease and its sequelae. *JAMA* 1991;**266**:2581–2586.
42. Wølner-Hanssen P, Eschenbach DA, Paavonen J, et al. Decreased risk of symptomatic chlamydial pelvic inflammatory disease associated with oral contraceptive use. *JAMA* 1990;**263**:54–59.
43. Svensson L, Weström L, Mardh P-A. Contraceptives and acute salpingitis. *JAMA* 1987;**251**:2553–2555.
44. Wølner-Hansen P, Svensson L, Mardh P-A, et al. Laparoscopic findings and contraceptive use in women with signs and symptoms suggestive of acute salpingitis. *Obstet Gynecol* 1985;**66**:233–239.
45. Rubin GL, Ory HW, Layde PM. Oral contraceptives and pelvic inflammatory disease. *Am J Obstet Gynecol* 1982;**140**:630–635.
46. Koch ML. The bactericidal action of beta progesterone. *Am J Obstet Gynecol* 1950;**59**:168–171.
47. Morse SA, Fitzgerald TJ. Effect of progesterone on *Neisseria gonorrhoeae*. *Infect Immun* 1974;**10**:1370–1377.
48. Salit IE. The differential susceptibility of gonococcal opacity variants to sex hormones. *Can J Microbiol* 1982;**28**:301–306.
49. Fitzgerald TJ, Morse SA. Alterations of growth, infectivity, and viability of *Neisseria gonorrhoeae* by gonadal steroids. *Can J Microbiol* 1976;**22**:286–294.
50. Cross CE, Halliwell B, Borish ET, et al. Oxygen radicals and human disease. *Ann Intern Med* 1987;**107**:526–545.
51. Eschenbach DA. Epidemiology and diagnosis of acute pelvic inflammatory disease. *Obstet Gynecol* 1980;**55**:142(S).
52. Cunningham FG, Hauth JC, Gilstrap LC, Herbert WNP, Kappus S. The bacterial pathogenesis of acute pelvic inflammatory disease. *Obstet Gynecol* 1978;**52**:161.
53. Holtz F. Klinische studien uber die nicht tuberkulose salpingoophoritis. *Acta Obstet Gynecol* 1930;**10**(S):5.
54. Falk V. Treatment of acute nontuberculous salpingitis with antibiotics alone and in combination with glucocorticoids. *Acta Obstet Gynecol Scand* 1965;**44**(S-16):65.
55. Hundley JM, Diehl WK, Baggott JW. Bacteriologic studies in salpingitis with special reference to gonococcal viability. *Am J Obstet Gynecol* 1950;**60**:97.
56. Jacobson L, Weström L. Objectivized diagnosis of acute pelvic inflammatory disease. *Am J Obstet Gynecol* 1969;**105**:1088.

57. Lip J, Burgoyne X. Cervical and peritoneal bacterial flora associated with salpingitis. *Obstet Gynecol* 1966;**28**:561.
58. Hedberg E, Spetz SV. Acute salpingitis: Views on prognosis and treatment. *Acta Obstet Gynecol Scand* 1958;**37**:131.
59. Thompson SE, Hager WD, Wong KH, et al. The microbiology and therapy of acute pelvic inflammatory disease in hospitalized patients. *Am J Obstet Gynecol* 1980;**136**:179.
60. Rendtorff RC, Curran JC, Chandler RW, et al. Economic consequences of gonorrhea in women. *J Am Vener Dis Assoc* 1974;**1**:40.
61. Eschenbach DA, Holmes KK. Acute pelvic inflammatory disease: Current concepts of pathogenesis, etiology, and management. *Clin Obstet Gynecol* 1975;**18**:35.
62. McCormack WM, Nowroozi K, Alpert S. Acute pelvic inflammatory disease: Characteristics of patients with gonococcal infection and evaluation of their response to treatment with aqueous procaine penicillin G and spectinomycin hydrochloride. *Sex Transm Dis* 1977;**4**:125.
63. Sweet RL, Mills J, Hadley WK, et al. Use of laparoscopy to determine the microbiologic etiology of acute salpingitis. *Am J Obstet Gynecol* 1979; **1334**:68.
64. Toth A, O'Leary WM, Ledger WJ. Evidence for microbial transfer by spermatozoa. *Obstet Gynecol* 1982;**59**:556–559.
65. Carney FE, Taylor-Robinson D. Growth and effect of *Neisseria gonorrhoeae* in organ cultures. *Br J Vener Dis* 1973;**49**:435.
66. McGee ZA, Johnson AP, Taylor-Robinson D. Pathogenic mechanisms of *Neisseria gonorrhoeae*. Observations on damage to human fallopian tubes in organ culture by gonococci of colony type 1 or type 4. *J Infect Dis* 1981;**143**:413–422.
67. Melly MA, Gregg CR, McGee ZA. Studies of toxicity of *Neisseria gonorrhoeae* for human fallopian tube mucosa. *J Infect Dis* 1981;**143**:423–431.
68. Melley MA, McGee ZA, Rosenthal RS. Ability of monomeric peptidoglycan fragments from *Neisseria gonorrhoeae* to damage human fallopian tube mucosa. *J Infect Dis* 1984;**149**:378–386.
69. Mulks MH, Plaut AG. IgA protease production as a characteristic distinguishing pathogenic from harmless Neisseria. *N Engl J Med* 1978;**299**:973–976.
70. Grifo JA, Jeremias J, Ledger WE, et al. Interferon-gamma in the diagnosis and pathogenesis of pelvic inflammatory disease. *Am J Obstet Gynecol* 1989;**160**:26–30.
71. Draper DL, James JF, Brooks GF, Sweet RL. Comparison of virulence markers of peritoneal-fallopian tube and endocervical *Neisseria gonorrhoeae* isolates from women with acute salpingitis. *Infect Immun* 1980;**27**:882.
72. Draper DL, James JF, Hadley WK, Sweet RL. Auxotypes and antibiotic susceptibilities of *Neisseria gonorrhoeae* from women with acute salpingitis. Comparison with gonococci causing uncomplicated genital tract infections in women. *Sex Transm Dis* 1981;**8**:43.
73. Draper DL, Donegan EA, James JF, Sweet RL, Brooks GF. Scanning electron microscopy of attachment of *Neisseria gonorrhoeae* colony phenotypes to surfaces of human genital epithelia. *Am J Obstet Gynecol* 1980;**138**:818.
74. Kellog DS Jr, et al. *Neisseria gonorrhoeae*: I. Virulence genetically linked to colony variations. *J Bact* 1963;**85**:1274–1279.

75. Kellog DS Jr, et al. *Neisseria gonorrhoeae*: II. Colonical variation and pathogenecity during 35 months in vitro. *J Bact* 1968;**90**:596–605.
76. Eilard ET, Brorsson J-E, Hanmark B, Forssman L. Isolation of chlamydia in acute salpingitis. *Scand J Infect Dis* 1976;**9**(S):82.
77. Mardh P-A, Ripa T, Svensson L, et al. *Chlamydia trachomatis* infection in patients with acute salpingitis. *N Engl J Med* 1977;**298**:1377.
78. Treharne JD, Ripa KT, Mardh P-A, et al. Antibodies to *Chlamydia trachomatis* in acute salpingitis. *Br J Vener Dis* 1979;**5**:26.
79. Paavonen J, Saikku P, Vesterinen E, Ako K. *Chlamydia trachomatis* in acute salpingitis. *Br J Vener Dis* 1979;**55**:703.
80. Paavonen J. *Chlamydia trachomatis* in acute salpingitis. *Am J Obstet Gynecol* 1980;**138**:957.
81. Mardh P-A, Lind I, Svensson L, et al. Antibodies to *Chlamydia trachomatis*, *Mycoplasma hominis* and *Neisseria gonorrhoeae* in serum from patients with acute salpingitis. *Br J Vener Dis* 1981;**57**:125.
82. Ripa KT, Svensson L, Treharne JD, et al. *Chlamydia trachomatis* infection in patients with laparoscopically verified acute salpingitis: results of isolation and antibody determinations. *Am J Obstet Gynecol* 1980;**138**:960.
83. Gjonnaess H, Dalaker K, Anestad G, et al. Pelvic inflammatory disease: Etiological studies with emphasis on chlamydial infection. *Obstet Gynecol* 1982;**59**:550–555.
84. Møller BR, Mardh P-A, Ahrons S, Nussler E. Infection with *Chlamydia trachomatis*, *Mycoplasma hominis*, and *Neisseria gonorrhoeae* in patients with acute pelvic inflammatory disease. *Sex Transm Dis* 1981;**8**:198–202.
85. Osser S, Poersson K. Epidemiology and serodiagnostic aspects of chlamydial salpingitis. *Obstet Gynecol* 1982;**59**:206–209.
86. Svensson L, Weström L, Ripa KT, et al. Differences in some clinical laboratory parameters in acute salpingitis related to culture and serologic findings. *Am J Obstet Gynecol* 1980;**138**:1017.
87. Bowie WR, Jones H. Acute inflammatory disease in outpatients: Association with *Chlamydia trachomatis* and *Neisseria gonorrhoeae*. *Ann Intern Med* 1981;**95**:686–688.
88. Kiviat NB, Wølner-Hanssen P, Peterson M, et al. Localization of *Chlamydia trachomatis* infection by direct immunofluorescence and culture in pelvic inflammatory disease. *Am J Obstet Gynecol* 1986;**154**:865–873.
89. Landers DV, Wølner-Hanssen P, Paavonen J et al. Combination antimicrobial therapy in the treatment of acute pelvic inflammatory disease. *Am J Obstet Gynecol* 1991;**164**:849–858.
90. Punnonen R, Terho P, Nikkanen V, et al. Chlamydial serology in infertile women by immunofluorescence. *Fertil Steril* 1979;**31**:656.
91. Henry–Suchet J, Loffredo V, Sarfaty D: *Chlamydia trachomatis* and mycoplasma research by laparoscopy in cases of pelvic inflammatory disease and in cases of tubal obstruction. *Am J Obstet Gynecol* 1980;**138**:1022.
92. Brunham RS, MacLean IW, Binns B, et al. *Chlamydia trachomatis*: Its role in tubal infertility. *J Infect Dis* 1985;**152**:1275.
93. Brunham RS, Binns B, McDowell J, et al. *Chlamydia trachomatis* infection in women with ectopic pregnancy. *Obstet Gynecol* 1986;**67**:722.
94. Svensson L, Mardh P-A, Ahlgren M, et al. Ectopic pregnancy and antibiotics to *Chlamydia trachomatis*. *Fertil Steril* 1985;**44**:313.

95. Hartford SL, Silva PD, diZerega GS, et al. Serologic evidence of prior chlamydial infection in patients with tubal ectopic pregnancy and contralateral tubal disease. *Fertil Steril* 1987;**47**:118.

96. Hutchinson GR, Taylor–Robinson D, Dourmashkin RR. Growth and effect of chlamydia in human and bovine oviduct cultures. *Br J Vener Dis* 1979;**55**:194.

97. Ripa KR, Møller BR, Mardh P-A, et al. Experimental acute salpingitis in grivet monkeys provoked by *Chlamydia trachomatis*. *Acta Pathol Microbiol Scand* 1979;**87**:65.

98. White HJ, Rank RG, Soloff BL, Barron AL: Experimental chlamydial salpingitis in immunosuppressed guinea pigs infected in the genital tract with agent of guinea pig inclusion conjunctivitis. *Infect Immun* 1979;**26**:573.

99. Sweet RL, Banks J, Sung M, Donegan E, Schachter J. Experimental chlamydial salpingitis in the guinea pig. *Am J Obstet Gynecol* 1980;**138**:952.

100. Swenson CE, Donegan E, Schachter J. *Chlamydia trachomatis*-induced salpingitis in mice. *J Infect Dis* 1983;**148**:1101–1107.

101. Swenson CE, Schachter J. Infertility as a consequence of chlamydial infection of the upper genital tract in female mice. *Sex Transm Dis* 1984;**11**:64–67.

102. Mardh P-A, Møller BR, Paavonen J: Chlamydial infection of the female genital tract with emphasis on pelvic inflammatory disease. A review of Scandinavian studies. *Sex Transm Dis* 1981;**8**(S):140–155.

103. Patton DL, Halbert SA, Kuo CC, Wang SP, Holmes KK. Host response to primary *Chlamydia trachomatis* infection of the fallopian tube in pig-tailed monkeys. *Fertil Steril* 1983;**40**:829–840.

104. Patton DL, Kuo CC, Wang SP, Halbert SA. Distal obstruction induced by repeated *Chlamydia trachomatis* salpingeal infection in pig-tailed mocaques. *J Infect Dis* 1987;**155**:1292–1299.

105. Patton DL, Landers DV, Schachter J. Experimental *Chlamydia trachomatis* salpingitis in mice: Initial studies on the characterization of the leukocyte response to chlamydia infection. *J Infect Dis* 1989;**159**:1105–1110.

106. Patton DL, Wang SP, Sternfield MD, et al. Chlamydial infection of subcutaneous fimbrial tansplants in cynomolgus and rhesus monkeys. *J Infect Dis* 1987;**155**:229–235.

107. Patton DL, Kuo CC. Histopathology of *Chlamydia trachomatis* salpingitis after primary and repeated infections in the monkey subcutaneous pocket model. *J Reprod Fertil* 1989;**85**:647–656.

108. Morrison RP, Lyng K, Caldwell HD. Chlamydial disease pathogenesis: Ocular hypersensitivity elicted by a genus-specific 57-KD protein. *J Exp Med* 1989; **169**:663–675.

109. Grayston JT, Wang SP, Yeh L-J, Kuo CC. Importance of reinfection in the pathogenesis of trachoma. *Rev Infect Dis* 1985;**7**:717–725.

110. Møller BR, Weström L, Ahrons S, et al. *Chlamydia trachomatis* infection of the fallopian tubes: Histological findings in two patients. *Br J Vener Dis* 1979;**55**:422–428.

111. Wager EA, Schachter J, Bavoil P, Stephens RS. Differential human serologic response to two 60,000 molecular weight *Chlamydia trachomatis* antigens. *J Infect Dis* 1990;**162**:922–927.

112. Brunham RC, Peeling R, Maclean I, et al. Postabortal *Chlamydia trachomatis* salpingitis: Correlating risk with antigenic-specific serological responses and with neutralization. *J Infect Dis* 1987;**155**:749–755.

113. Witkin SS, Jeremias J, Toth M, Ledger WJ. Cell-mediated immune response to the recombinant 57-KD heat-shock protein of *Chlamydia trachomatis* in women with salpingitis. *J Infect Dis* 1993;**167**:1379–1383.

114. Patton DL, Cosgrove Sweeney YT, Kuo C-C. Demonstration of delayed hypersensitivity in *Chlamydia trachomatis* salpingitis in monkeys. A pathogenic mechanism of tubal damage. *J Infect Dis* 1994;**169**:680–683.

115. Morrison RP, Belland RJ, Lyngk, Caldwell HD. Chlamydial disease pathogenesis. The 57-KD hypersensitivity antigen in a stress response protein. *J Exp Med* 1989;**170**:1271–1283.

116. Andrews FT. Notes on causes of salpingitis. *Am J Obstet Gynecol* 1940;**49**:177.

117. Chow AW, Malkasian KL, Marshall Jr, et al. The bacteriology of acute pelvic inflammatory disease. *Am J Obstet Gynecol* 1975;**122**:876.

118. Cunningham FG, Hauth JC, Strong JD, et al. Evaluation of tetracycline or penicillin and ampicillin for the treatment of acute pelvic inflammatory disease. *N Engl J Med* 1977;**296**:1380.

119. Monif GRG, Welkos SL, Baer H, et al. Cul de sac isolates from patients with endometritis, salpingitis, peritonitis and gonococcal endocervicitis. *Am J Obstet Gynecol* 1976;**126**:158.

120. Sweet RL, Draper D, Hadley WK. Etiology of acute salpingitis: Influence of episode number and duration of symptoms. *Obstet Gynecol* 1981;**58**:62.

121. Soper DE, Brockwell NJ, Dalton HP. False-positive cultures of the cul-de-sac associated with culdocentesis in patients undergoing elective laparoscopy. *Obstet Gynecol* 1991;**77**:134–138.

122. Sweet RL, Schachter J, Landers DV, et al. Treatment of hospitalized patients with acute pelvic inflammatory disease: Comparison of cefotetan plus doxycycline and cefoxitin plus doxycycline. *Am J Obstet Gynecol* 1988;**158**:736–743.

123. Landers DV, Wølner-Hanssen P, Paavonen J, et al. Combination antimicrobial therapy in the treatment of acute pelvic inflammatory disease. *Am J Obstet Gynecol* 1991;**164**:849–858.

124. Paavonen J, Teisala K, Heinonnen PK, et al. Microbiological and histopathological findings in acute pelvic inflammatory disease. *Br J Obstet Gynecol* 1987;**94**:454–460.

125. Brunham RC, Binns B, Guijon F, et al. Etiology and outcome of acute pelvic inflammatory disease. *J Infect Dis* 1988;**158**:510–517.

126. Paavonen J, Valtonen VV, Kasper DL, et al. Serological evidence for the role of *Bacteroides fragilis* and enterobacteriaceae in the pathogenesis of acute pelvic inflammatory diasese. *Lancet* 1981;**1**:293–295.

127. Curtis AH. Bacteriology and pathology of fallopian tubes removed at operation. *Surg Gynecol Obstet* 1921;**33**:621.

128. Eschenbach DA, Holmes KK. Gonococcal pelvic inflammatory disease (Letter). *Am J Obstet Gynecol* 1977;**129**:710–711.

129. Monif GRG. Gonococcal endometritis-salpingitis-peritonitis. *Am J Obstet Gynecol* 1977;**129**:711–714.

130. Phiefer TA, Forsyth PS, Durfee MA, et al. Nonspecific vaginitis: Role of *Haemophilus vaginalis* and treatment with metronidazole. *N Engl J Med* 1978;**298**:1429.

131. Holmes KK, Speigel C, Amsel R, et al. Nonspecific vaginosis. *Scand J Infect Dis* 1981;**26**(S):110.

132. Spiegal CA, Amsel R, Eschenbach DA, et al. Anaerobic bacteria in non-specific vaginitis. *N Engl J Med* 1980;**303**:601.
133. Taylor E, Barlow D, Blackwell AL, Phillips I. *Gardnerella vaginalis*, anaerobes and vaginal discharge. *Lancet* 1982;**2**:1376–1379.
134. Spiegal CA, Eschenbach DA, Amsel R, Holmes KK. Curved anaerobic bacteria in bacterial (nonspecific) vaginosis and their response to therapy. *J Infect Dis* 1983;**148**:817.
135. Paavonen J, Teisala K, Heinonnen PK, et al. Microbiological and histopathological findings in acute pelvic inflammatory disease. *Brit J Obstet Gynecol* 1987;**94**:454–460.
136. Eschenbach DA, Hillier S, Critchlow C, et al. Diagnosis and clinical manifestations of bacterial vaginosis. *Am J Obstet Gynecol* 1988;**158**:819–828.
137. Soper DE, Brockwell NJ, Dalton HP, Johnson D. Observations concerning the microbial etiology of acute salpingitis. *Am J Obstet Gynecol* 1994;**170**:1008–1017.
138. Eschenbach DA. Acute pelvic inflammatory disease. *Urol Clin North Am* 1984;**11**:65–81.
139. Goldacre MJ, Watt B, London N, et al. Vaginal microbial flora in normal young women. *Br Med J* 1979;**1**:1450–1453.
140. Bartlett JG, Onderdonk AB, Drude E, et al. Quantitative bacteriology of the vaginal flora. *J Infect Dis* 1977;**126**:271.
141. Sparks RA, Purrier BG, Watt PJ, Elstein M. Bacteriological colonization of uterine cavity; role of tailed intrauterine contraceptive devices. *Br Med J* 1981;**282**:1189–1191.
142. Skangalis M, Mahoney CJ, O'Leary WM. Microbial presence in the uterine cavity as affected by varieties of intrauterine contraceptive devices. *Fertil Steril* 1982;**37**:263–269.
143. Taylor ES, McMillan JH, Greer BE, Drogemueller W, Thompson HE. The intrauterine device and tubo-ovarian abscesses. *Am J Obstet Gynecol* 1975;**123**:338.
144. Ober WB, Sobrero AJ, de Chabon AB, Goodman J. Polyethylene intrauterine contraceptive device. Endometrial changes following long-term use. *JAMA* 1970;**212**:765–769.
145. Landers DV, Sweet RL. Tubo-ovarian abscess: Contemporary approach to management. *Rev Infect Dis* 1983;**5**:876–884.
146. Lemcke R, Csonka GW. Antibodies against pleuropneumonia-like organisms in patients with salpingitis. *Br J Vener Dis* 1962;**38**:212–217.
147. Mardh P-A, Weström L. Tubal and cervical cultures in acute salpingitis with special reference to *Mycoplasma hominis* and T-strain mycoplasmas. *Br J Vener Dis* 1970;**46**:169.
148. Møller BR. The role of mycoplasmas in the upper genital tract of women. *Sex Transm Dis* 1983;**10**(S):281–284.
149. Mardh P-A, Lind I, Svensson L, et al. Antibodies to *Chlamydia trachomatis*, *Mycoplasma hominis* and *Neisseria gonorrhoeae* in serum from patients with acute salpingitis. *Br J Vener Dis* 1981;**57**:125–129.
150. Taylor–Robinson D, Carney FE. Growth and effect of mycoplasmas in fallopian tube organ cultures. *Br J Vener Dis* 1974;**50**:212.
151. Hare MJ, Barnes CFJ. Fallopian tube organ culture in the investigation of bacteroides as a cause of pelvic inflammatory disease, in Philips I, Collier J

(eds): *Metronidazole: Royal Society of Medicine International Congress and Symposium Series No. 18.* London, Academic Press, 1979.

152. Taylor–Robinson D, McCormack WM. The genital mycoplasmas. *N Engl J Med* 1980;**302**:1003.

153. Møller BR, Freundt EA, Black FT, et al. Experimental infection of the genital tract of female grivet monkeys for *Mycoplasma hominis*. *Infect Immun* 1978;**20**:248.

154. Mardh P-A, Weström L, vanMecklenberg C, et al. Studies on ciliated epithelia of the human genital tract. I. Swelling of the cilia of fallopian tube epithelium in organ cultures infected with *Mycoplasma hominis*. *Br J Vener Dis* 1976;**52**:52.

155. Paavonen J, Teisala K, Heinonnen PK, et al. Endometritis and acute salpingitis associated with *Chlamydia trachomatis* and herpes simplex virus type two. *Obstet Gynecol* 1985;**65**:288–291.

156. Lehtinen M, Rantala I, Teisala K, et al. Detection of herpes simplex virus in women with acute pelvic inflammatory disease. *J Infect Dis* 1985;**152**:78–82.

157. Walters MD, Eddy CA, Gibbs RS, et al. Antibodies to *Chlamydia trachomatis* and the risk of tubal pregnancy. *Am J Obstet Gynecol* 1988,**159**:942–946.

158. Chow JM, Yonekura ML, Richwald GA, et al. The association between *Chlamydia trachomatis* and ectopic pregnancy: A matched-pair, case-control study. *JAMA* 1990;**263**:3164–3167.

4
Diagnosis of Pelvic Inflammatory Disease

PÅL WØLNER-HANSSEN

Pelvic inflammatory disease (PID) is difficult to diagnose. Symptoms and signs associated with PID are common for different diseases and vary from case to case. Without invasive procedures, the organs of interest are invisible and indirectly palpable. The result is that we sometimes misdiagnose PID in healthy women (overdiagnosis). Sometimes we think women with acute PID are healthy (underdiagnosis), and sometimes we diagnose PID in women who have other diseases (misdiagnosis). Overdiagnosis may lead to inappropriate hospital care, antibiotic treatment, and surgery. Underdiagnosis may lead to delayed antibiotic treatment with increased risk for complications, including tubo-ovarian abscess, infertility, and later, ectopic pregnancy. Misdiagnosis may result in delay of appropriate treatment of other diseases, including appendicitis and ectopic pregnancy.

Those concerned with acute gynecology are familiar with the problems of PID diagnostics. Most authors agree that clinical diagnoses of PID cannot be relied on. Nevertheless, studies are still published in which presumed diagnoses of PID were not confirmed by laparoscopy. In clinical practice, laparoscopy will probably not be routine in the foreseeable future. The reason is that laparoscopy is an invasive, expensive, and potentially harmful procedure.

In this chapter, current knowledge of the diagnostic value of different clinical, laboratory, and surgical parameters will be discussed.

Clinical Manifestations

Symptoms

Lower abdominal pain is a principal symptom of acute PID. The intensity of pain is variable. Some women have excruciating pain; others have no pain at all. The prevalence of abdominal pain among women with PID is unknown, because most PID studies use this symptom as a mandatory entry criterion.

Good analyses of the character of abdominal pain caused by PID are not available. The personal impression of this author is that abdominal pain associated with PID usually is continuous, sometimes with crampy exacerbations. In PID, the pain is usually bilateral. Women with appendicitis more frequently have isolated right lower abdominal pain than those with PID ($p < 0.001$).[1] When the infection has spread to the liver capsule (perihepatitis or "Fitz–Hugh–Curtis syndrome"), severe right-upper abdominal pain may occur. Duration of pain before presentation to the hospital also has differential diagnostic value. On average, women with PID have had pain twice as long as those having appendicitis (median 48 h vs. median 21 h).[1] Nine of ten patients with acute salpingitis have had pain for less than 3 weeks.[2] Women with acute PID may have had pain for a longer period. However, one should seriously consider other conditions for women with pain for more than a month. In a recent, excellent review, Kahn and coworkers[3] analyzed available literature for the diagnostic value of clinical symptoms. Abdominal pain for more than 4 days was the most sensitive (76%), but the least specific (46%) predictor of chlamydial salpingitis.[4] Abdominal pain for 4 to 7 days was a more specific (89%) but less sensitive (33%) predictor.[4]

Patients with acute PID may report several nonspecific genital and extragenital symptoms, including discharge, abnormal bleeding, nausea and vomiting, diarrhea, dysuria, and frequency. Several studies have reported relationships between these findings and acute PID. Pain in the rectum, dysuria/frequency, irregular menses, and fever/chills have a specificity above 60% and a sensitivity below 55% for PID.[3] Among women with acute abdominal pain, vomiting is not a predictor of salpingitis.[5] However, compared with women having appendicitis, those with PID were significantly less likely to report vomiting.[1]

Endometritis is one cause of abnormal bleeding. We studied 763 randomly selected women attending a sexually transmitted disease (STD) clinic in Seattle (Wølner-Hanssen et al., unpublished data). Among nonusers of oral contraceptives, those reporting heavier last menstrual bleeding than normal tended to be infected with *Chlamydia trachomatis* (odds ratio = 2.6, $p = 0.001$), *Neisseria gonorrhoeae* (odds ratio = 2.1, $p = 0.008$), or bacterial vaginosis (odds ratio = 1.9, $p = 0.001$). Those reporting metrorrhagia also tended to have *C. trachomatis* infection (odds ratio = 2.0, $p = 0.04$). In women using oral contraceptives, menorrhagia or metrorrhagia did not correlate with genital infections. That is, abnormal bleeding not attributable to oral contraceptive use may be a manifestation of endometritis. We do not know how often women with abnormal bleeding and chlamydial or gonococcal infection also have salpingitis.

Abnormal vaginal discharge may be a symptom of genital infection. However, a history of abnormal discharge was not significantly associated with PID in any of four studies concerned with the symptom.[3]

Signs

On pelvic examination, adnexal tenderness, uterine tenderness, and cervical motion tenderness are nonspecific signs frequently occurring in acute PID. In most studies, adnexal tenderness and cervical motion tenderness are inclusion criteria. Therefore, we do not know how accurate these signs predict PID. In the only study reporting on the associations of adnexal tenderness and cervical motion tenderness with PID, the associations were not significant.[6] Adnexal tenderness is usually bilateral but may be unilateral.[1] Adnexal masses may be due to tubo-ovarian abscesses, peri-appendiceal abscesses, ovarian tumors, or cysts. It is difficult to distinguish between these conditions with palpating hands. Nevertheless, presence of adnexal mass had a positive predictive value of 75%, while absence of pelvic mass had a negative predictive value of 28% for acute salpingitis in one study of women with chlamydial infection.[4]

Fever (body temperature ≥38°C) is an uncommon sign of PID. Only 20% of women with chlamydial salpingitis have fever at the initial examination.[4] Of women infected with *C. trachomatis* and with clinical evidence of acute PID, but without confirmation of acute salpingitis, 21% have fever.[4] In women with acute salpingitis of any etiology, only one-third have a temperature above 38°C. The positive predictive value of fever was 75%, and the negative predictive value of no fever 28% in the study of chlamydial positive women.[4]

Birth Control Methods and Clinical Manifestations of PID

Several reports have shown that different birth control methods may alter the natural course and manifestations of acute PID. Most reports have concerned oral contraceptive use. Among women infected with *C. trachomatis*, oral contraceptive users had five times less risk of acute PID compared with users of no methods.[7] Among women infected with *N. gonorrhoeae* there was no relationship between oral contraceptive use and acute PID. Oral contraceptive users with signs and symptoms of acute PID, less often had laparoscopic signs of acute salpingitis than users of no birth control method.[8] We found this trend among women infected with *C. trachomatis* and among those infected with *N. gonorrhoeae*. Oral contraceptive users with salpingitis had milder tubal changes than nonusers with salpingitis.[9] Among women with chlamydial salpingitis, none of 38 oral contraceptive users had perihepatitis. One-sixth of intrauterine device (IUD) users and one-fifth of those using no method or barrier method had perihepatitis.[10] These findings resulted in speculations that oral contraceptive use may tend to cause asymptomatic or "silent" chlamydial PID.[11] Patients and clinicians may not recognize asymptomatic PID. The infection may then run its natural course, leaving the unwitting patient infertile.

However, no available data confirm these speculations. Whether oral contraceptive users tend to develop particularly mild clinical manifestations of chlamydial PID is unknown.

Many believe that use of an IUD increases the risk of developing acute PID. Use of an IUD significantly predicted PID in one of three studies.[3] However, there is no evidence that use of the now available IUDs alter manifestations of acute PID.

Tubal ligation protects women against acute salpingitis. In one report, the author claimed that none of 3,500 women who had undergone laparoscopic sterilization had been admitted with the diagnosis of acute PID.[12] After sterilization, the lumen of the distal part of the tube has no connection with the uterine lumen. Therefore, there is little risk for the distal part becoming involved in PID. The lumen of the proximal stump connects with the uterine cavity. In sterilized women, endometritis might therefore spread into the proximal stump and cause "proximal stump salpingitis" (PSS). The proximal stump may then be erythematous, edematous, and pus may come out from its distal end. Case reports, but no systematic study on proximal stump salpingitis are available.[13]

In women with signs and symptoms of PID, a history of tubal ligation does not a priori rule out the disease.

Laboratory Tests

Urine Tests

The most important laboratory test for women with acute pelvic pain is a rapid and sensitive pregnancy test. Acute PID is unusual in pregnant women. In most cases, the clinician can rule out PID if the pregnancy test is positive. However, tubo-ovarian abscesses may occur during pregnancy.[14]

Blood Tests

The most important laboratory test among those with acute pelvic pain and a negative pregnancy test is measurement of C-reactive protein (CRP) level. The sensitivity and specificity of CRP for acute PID range from 74% to 93%, and from 67% to 81%, respectively, depending upon whether a cut-off point of 20mg/L or 10mg/L was used.[15,16] Of 115 women with a presumed diagnosis of acute pID, 78 had acute salpingitis by laparoscopy or laparotomy.[17] Using a cut-off point of 6mg/L, CRP had an impressing positive predictive value of 98% and a negative predictive value of 98% for a visual diagnosis of acute salpingitis. The CRP-level may also be predictive of the severity of the inflammation (see below).

Other often-used tests are the erythrocyte sedimentation rate (ESR), and the white blood cell count (WBC). According to multivariate analyses of data from 616 women who underwent laparoscopy, elevated ESR (>15 mm/h) is a strong predictor of acute salpingitis.[5] The sensitivity of elevated ESR is between 75% and 81%, and the specificity between 25% and 68% for acute PID.[4,15,18] Among women with chlamydial infection, the positive predictive value of elevated ESR (>15 mm/h) is 87%.[4] Only 44% of women with acute chlamydial salpingitis have elevated WBC. Of women with chlamydial infection and pelvic pain, but without confirmed salpingitis, 32% had elevated WBC. Women with severe salpingitis more often have elevated ESR and WBC than those with mild salpingitis.[18]

Serum IgG antibodies to *C. trachomatis* are common among women with laparoscopically verified salpingitis.[19] Also infertile women with scarred tubes due to previous salpingitis,[20] and women with mucopurulent cervicitis, often have chlamydial antibodies.[19] It has been claimed that serum IgA antibodies to *C. trachomatis* predict chlamydial infection better than cultures do.[21] This claim has not been substantiated in the literature. It is therefore not worthwhile to determine chlamydial antibodies in routine care of patients with suspected PID.

Evaluation of Cervical and Vaginal Contents

Presence of pathogens in the lower genital tract is a prerequisite for acute PID. It is therefore of interest to look for signs of inflammation in the cervix and vagina in women with pelvic pain.

Grossly purulent cervical mucus (mucopus) reflects a high concentration of polymorphonuclear leukocytes (PMNs) in the mucus. In less clear cases, Gram stained mucus smears may be used to identify PMNs under the microscope. Of women with ≥10 PMNs per 1200 × field of Gram-stained cervical mucus, 85% had infection with *C. trachomatis*.[22] Only 20% of those with fewer than 10 cells per field had chlamydial infection ($p < 0.01$). Among women with 10 or more PMNs per microscopy field *and/or* purulent cervical discharge, 38% have chlamydial infection.[23] With increasing concentration of PMNs in the mucus, the chance of a positive *C. trachomatis* culture increases. The sensitivity of cervical Gram stains for chlamydial infection decreases from 91% to 38% and the specificity increases from 65% to 89% with increasing cut-off point from 5 or more to 15 or more PMNs.[24] This means that it may be worthwhile to examine cervical Gram stains to screen for *C. trachomatis*, at least in high-prevalence populations such as women with acute PID. However, there are no good data available to show an association between cervical mucopus and acute PID. The one time it was studied, cervical discharge did not predict PID.[6]

Many clinicians examine vaginal smears mixed with isotone saline solution (wet mounts) by microscopy to screen women for pelvic infection. Higher numbers of leukocytes than of vaginal epithelial cells in random microscopy fields is thought to predict infection. However, no controlled studies are available to support this belief. In the original work by Weström, leukocytes outnumbered all other cellular elements in the smears of 92% of women in whom PID could not be confirmed.[2] There is no association between chlamydial infection and a leukocyte-dominated wet mount.[25] Moreover, macroscopic purulent vaginal discharge, albeit being a sensitive sign (87%), is nonspecific for PID (25%).[4]

Microbiology

Treatment has to start before culture results are available in cases of suspected PID. Broad spectrum antibiotic regimens cover most microorganisms involved in PID. Nevertheless, one should perform a microbiological work-up. The culture results might explain treatment failures, add weight to the recommendation of partner treatment, and educate the patient about her disease. Minimal microbiological work-up is cervical culture for *N. gonorrhoeae* and culture or antigen detection test for *C. trachomatis*. Cervical cultures for anaerobic or facultative organisms, or for *M. hominis*, are of little value. These microorganisms are present in the lower genital tract of many healthy women, and the culture results do not reflect upper genital tract flora. Some investigators aspirate endometrial material for culture in patients with PID. This author and other authors do not believe that endometrial cultures reflect upper genital microbiology any better than cervical cultures. One can never rule out contamination of endometrial specimens by the vaginal flora. In some cases, however, endometrial cultures identify microorganisms not found in the cervical culture. In some cases, endometrial, but not cervical specimens may grow out *C. trachomatis*.

Culdocentesis

Peritoneal fluid is easy to get by culdocentesis. The fluid can be examined for leukocytes by microscopy, and for microorganisms by culture. Some clinicians regard the presence of leukocytes in the peritoneal fluid as a confirmation of pelvic infection, and attribute pathogens isolated to the pelvic infection. Weström found a higher concentration of WBC in the peritoneal fluids from women with acute salpingitis ($3.1–3.7 \times 10^{10}$/L) than in fluids from women with no infection ($0.3–1.3 \times 10^9$/L).[2] By contrast, Paavonen and coworkers found no significant association between presence of leukocytes in peritoneal fluid and laparoscopic evidence of salpingitis.[26] Sweet and coworkers compared specimens from the fallopian tubes taken via laparoscopy with cul-de-sac fluid taken via culdocentesis in patients with acute salpingitis.[27] The investigators isolated microorganisms more often from the culdocentesis material than from the laparoscopy material. This study supported a concern that vaginal flora may contaminate culdocentesis material. Therefore, this author does not recommend culdocentesis in routine PID work-up.

Laparoscopy

Swedish investigators introduced laparoscopy for the diagnosis of acute salpingitis in the 1950s. The method has now gained general acceptance as the "gold standard" for salpingitis diagnosis. Many European clinicians use laparoscopy routinely in cases of suspected PID. United States physicians have been more restrictive to laparoscopy for acute PID. However, some U.S. investigators use the method for research purposes.

Jacobson and Weström[18] formalized laparoscopic criteria for acute salpingitis. For a diagnosis of salpingitis, the fallopian tubes should be erythematous and edematous. However, tubal erythema and edema are common findings during normal menstrual periods. Therefore, at least one of the following signs must be present: pus coming from the distal tubal os or present inside the tube (pyosalpinx), fresh (easily breakable) periadnexal adhesions, and sticky exudate on the tubal surface. Using these criteria, Jacobson and Weström[18] confirmed salpingitis in only 65% of women initially thought to have acute PID. Other investigations later confirmed these results. In a Seattle study, we identified salpingitis in 79 (71%) of 112 patients thought to have acute PID (Wølner-Hanssen and coworkers, unpublished data).

To grade tubal inflammation during laparoscopy of women with salpingitis, one should look for the following: presence and extension of fresh adhesions involving the tubes, patency of the distal tubal os (fimbria intact, phimotic, or retracted to shut off the distal os), and enlargement of the tubal diameter. Table 4.1 shows the criteria for grading salpingitis as mild, moderate, and severe, as described by Jacobson and Weström. These criteria may not be perfect, but are the only ones shown to correlate with later fertility.

According to the unique follow-up study by Weström,[28] tubal infertility following one episode of mild, moderate, and severe salpingitis was 2.6%, 13%, and 28.6%, respectively. The degree of tubal inflammation is therefore important information for the patient. Without laparoscopy, tubal damage vaguely can be predicted. In Seattle, we studied correlations between tubal alterations and selected clinical and laboratory findings in 79 women with acute salpingitis (Wølner-Hanssen and coworkers, unpublished data). Mean ESR correlated significantly with the diameter of the

TABLE 4.1. Laparoscopic criteria for severity of salpingitis.*

Mild	Tubes freely moveable and with open abdominal ostia.
Moderate	Tubes are not freely moveable; patency of abdominal ostia uncertain.
Severe	Pelvoperitonitis and/or abscess formation[‡]

*If discrepancy between sides, the patient is classified according to the mildest side.
[‡] Includes pyosalpinx.
Source: Ref. 18.

largest fallopian tube ($p < 0.001$). Other variables studied included duration of abdominal pain, degree of tenderness on abdominal and pelvic examination, oral temperature, WBC, and CRP. None of these variables correlated with the tubal diameter. The presence of periadnexal adhesions or distal tubal occlusion did not correlate with any of the variables studied. Interestingly, the mean CRP level was significantly *lower* for women with adnexal adhesions (3.7 ± 3.9 mg/dL) than for those without adhesions (10.4 ± 4.8 mg/dL, $p = 0.0038$). This suggests that women with adhesions have longer standing infection. According to another laparoscopy study, the CRP level was 9.38 mg/dL (7.36–11.39) among those with severe PID, and 4.46 mg/dL (3.11–5.61) among those with mild PID.[29]

Laparoscopy is also a method to examine women with acute right-upper abdominal pain for perihepatitis. On laparoscopy, fibrinous, approximated adhesions between the anterior liver surface and the adjacent abdominal wall plus erythema of the surrounding peritoneum show acute perihepatitis. These adhesions are initially fragile, and may break during gas insufflation with the patient in the Trendelenburg position. A circular, fibrinous ridge on the liver surface, and an area of pin-point bleeding of the peritoneum on the corresponding abdominal wall may still reveal the perihepatic adhesion. Older cases of perihepatitis may have violin-string and filmy adhesions between the liver and the anterior abdominal wall.

The diagnostic value of laparoscopy has not been properly evaluated. Noteworthy is that we do not know the specificity and sensitivity of this "gold standard" for diagnosis of acute salpingitis. It is possible that sensitivity of the criteria used is not high. Many women with no other findings than reddened tubes, may in fact have salpingitis. Some women with normal-looking fallopian tubes may have endosalpingitis. For example, we have seen inflammatory responses in tubal biopsies and endotubal cytology smears from women in whom laparoscopy showed no salpingitis. Stacey and coworkers[30] performed laparoscopy in 23 women with lower abdominal pain and positive genital cultures for *C. trachomatis*. Laparoscopy revealed salpingitis in 11 of the 23 women. Four of the 12 women without salpingitis had *C. trachomatis* in the fallopian tubes. Endometrial histology revealed endometritis in two women without visible salpingitis; both of them had *C. trachomatis* isolated from the upper genital tract. This study also suggests that laparoscopy may miss some cases of upper genital tract infection. To test the accuracy of laparoscopy, we need another "gold standard." Sellors and coworkers[31] approached the problem by performing laparoscopy in women with acute abdominal pain, with or without a preliminary diagnosis of acute salpingitis. The investigators based a diagnosis of PID on laparoscopic findings together with histopathological findings (tubal and endometrial biopsies). Laparoscopic and histopathological findings did not correlate well. For example, laparoscopy missed half of those with biopsy-confirmed salpingitis. Of women thought by laparoscopy to have salpingitis, only 65% had histopathological evidence of salpingitis. A problem with these analyses is that the criteria for a histopathological diagnosis of salpingitis were arbitrarily chosen. Thus, when laparoscopy and histopathology do not correspond, it is difficult to decide which to rely on. As long as no other gold standard exists, it will be difficult to define the accuracy of laparoscopy. A gold standard simpler and cheaper than laparoscopy is desirable. It will be the challenge of the 1990s to identify a standard that satisfies the following requirement: "The ideal gold standard for PID would be the test that most closely correlates with acute and long-term clinical outcomes, assessed with prospective studies."[3]

There are several arguments for routine laparoscopy in women with acute lower abdominal pain. By inspecting the abdomen directly, one can prove the diagnosis and rule out other conditions. Correct diagnosis can shorten hospital stay, particularly in a case of normal-looking tubes. Direct visualization may prevent perforation of an otherwise undiagnosed acute appendicitis. By taking specimens from the tubes, one can identify microorganisms causing the infection. Culture results may guide antibiotic choices. One can evaluate the degree of tubal damage. This will permit the physician to inform the patient about her risks of future infertility and of tubal pregnancy. Tubo-ovarian abscesses can be treated by puncture and aspiration of pus. This may save some patients long-lasting hospital care and major surgery.

There are many arguments also against routine laparoscopy in cases of suspected PID. Laparoscopy is expensive. Many U.S. women with acute PID have no health insurance—a fact that might explain why most U.S. studies on PID are based on clinical criteria only. Laparoscopy is an invasive procedure requiring general anesthesia. The risks of laparoscopy include anesthetic complications and perforations of abdominal organs. The risk of dying by laparoscopy is approximately 1:10,000. Laparoscopy is cumbersome to arrange. The procedure needs to be done acutely and will utilize many personnel (in contrast to the simple prescription of antibiotics for an ambulatory case of possible PID). Many regard laparoscopy as an unnecessary procedure. Most women will receive antibiotics anyway, whether or not salpingitis is proven through the laparoscope.

It must be up to the practitioner to decide which of the arguments weigh heavier. For good PID research, however, laparoscopy is mandatory. Also, for cases of unclear, persisting or worsening pain, laparoscopy is important.

Endometrial Biopsy

In acute PID, an infection in the vagina/cervix has spread to the fallopian tubes via the endometrial cavity, causing endometritis. Investigators have used samples from the uterine cavity to identify endometritis by histopathological or microbiological methods. Above, we discussed endometrial culturing. Here, we will focus on endometrial biopsies.

An endometrial stripe biopsy is easy to obtain in the physicians's office. Any of the numerous available instruments for endometrial tissue sampling will do. In published studies, the Novack curette has often been used. An advantage with this curette is the relatively large specimen produced. A disadvantage with the Novack curette is the pain it may cause the unanesthetized patient. Some ambulatory patients will need a paracervical blockade. A less painful biopsy instrument is the Pipelle™ endometrial suction curette (Prodimed, Neuilly-en-Thelle, France).

The diagnosis of endometritis has been a matter of dispute among pathologists. For many years, pathologists defined endometritis by the presence of plasma cells in endometrial stroma. There was no agreement about the number of plasma cells required for a diagnosis of endometritis, however. Recently, inflammatory changes in endometrial biopsies from patients with acute abdominal pain who underwent laparoscopy, were analyzed.[32] The simultaneous presence of five or more PMNs per 400 × field in endometrial surface epithelium, and one or more plasma cells per 120 × field in endometrial stroma, strongly correlated with acute salpingitis and upper genital tract infection. This criterion had sensitivity of 78%, specificity of 95%, and positive predictive value of 97% for laparoscopic evidence of salpingitis. The negative predictive value of the criterion was only 67%. The low negative predictive value may be explained by a patchy inflammation of the endometrium. In some cases, the biopsy instrument will miss areas with inflammation.

Another criterion used in the study was "dense superficial stromal inflammation."[32] That is, more than 50% of superficial stromal tissue contains more than 50 leukocytes per 400 × field. This criterion had sensitivity of 81%, specificity of 90%, positive predictive value of 94%, and negative predictive value of 72% for acute salpingitis with pathogens isolated from the upper genital tract.

In summary, endometrial biopsy may be a useful diagnostic method in cases of suspected acute PID. Endometrial biopsy does not replace laparoscopy, but may be a valuable complement to laparoscopy. A disadvantage with endometrial biopsy is the delay of results. Under the best of circumstances, the result will not be available before a few days.

Ultrasonography

Normal fallopian tubes are often difficult to identify by ultrasonography. In one study, ultrasound criteria for PID included thickened, fluid-filled tubes alone or a thickened tube conglomerate with the ovary forming a tubo-ovarian complex.[33] The "golden standard" for PID in that study was presence of plasma cells in endometrial biopsies. The positive and negative predictive values for a finding of thickened tube was 100% and 95%, respectively. Polycystic ovaries were identified in all women with endometritis and in less than one-third of those without endometritis.[33] In another study, the investigators performed endovaginal ultrasonography with a 5-MHz transducer just before laparoscopy. They considered fallopian tubes abnormal if they were visibly distended by fluid, or if a thick-walled, echogenic, redundant tubular structure extended from the uterine cornua into the adnexal region.[34] Endovaginal ultrasonography correctly predicted 25 of 27 (93%) abnormal tubes. Ovarian enlargement and indistinct ovarian margins at ultrasonography predicted 19 of 21 cases with periovarian exudate and adhesions.

The goal of confirmatory tests of PID is not primarily to confirm what we already suspect. We also want to rule out other diseases (e.g., appendicitis, endometriosis) and to assess the severity of tubal damage. We cannot reach these goals with ultrasonography at this time, even when ultrasonography may be useful for appendicitis diagnosis.[35] Unless we perform laparoscopy, ultrasound may still be helpful in women who are difficult to examine. With ultrasonography tubo-ovarian abscesses can be ruled out. If tubo-ovarian abscesses are present, one may use ultrasonography to monitor regress of the abscesses during antibiotic therapy.

Diagnosis and Differential Diagnosis

The discussion above tried to demonstrate that no single symptom, sign, or laboratory test predicts PID with a high degree of certainty. Combinations of manifestations reported in the literature are either sensitive or specific, but not *both* sensitive *and* specific. For example, a combination of pelvic pain, adnexal tenderness, temperature >38°C, erythrocyte sedimentation rate >15 mm/h, and a palpable mass is 99% specific for salpingitis. Only one in six women with salpingitis has this combination, though.[36] Various signs and symptoms have different diagnostic value. Kahn and coworkers,[3] reviewing the available literature, found that the following clinical diagnostic indicators were important: abnormal vaginal discharge on examination, elevated CRP, elevated ESR, and endometritis by biopsy. Further indicators considered useful were: cervical motion tenderness, bilateral pain (as opposed to unilateral), negative pregnancy test, Gram negative intracellular diplococci in cervical mucus, and sonographic evidence of pelvic abscess.[3] There is no evidence that the WBC is useful for PID diagnostics.

When approaching a woman with acute abdominal pain, a thorough history is important. One should inquire in detail about location, duration, character, and pattern of abdominal pain. We can obtain important information from this inquiry. For example, unilateral right-sided pain may suggest appendicitis, ruptured ovarian cyst, twisted adnexa, or ectopic pregnancy. Instant onset of unilateral pain is typical for a ruptured ovarian cyst, ectopic pregnancy, or twisted adnexa. Gradual onset of pain over several hours, with pain moving from the epigastric area to the right-lower quadrant may suggest appendicitis. Gradually increasing pain in the right and left-lower abdominal quadrants is more typical for PID. One should ask patients for risk factors, including previous PID, symptomatic or new sexual partner, recently introduced IUD. To differentiate between infection and pregnancy, a thorough bleeding history may be helpful.

On physical examination, external abdominal palpation will help localize the disease process and detect peritonitis. Right-upper abdominal direct and rebound tenderness suggests perihepatitis. With bimanual pelvic examination one can identify adnexal and cervical motion tenderness and adnexal masses. Inspection of the cervix might reveal purulent cervical discharge, suggesting mucopurulent cervicitis. One should take the oral temperature. Fever is a reason to hospitalize a woman with acute abdominal pain. Mandatory laboratory tests are: *N gonorrhoeae* culture, *C. trachomatis* culture or antigen detection, pregnancy test, and serum C-reactive protein level.

Before we decide to treat a case of abdominal pain as an acute PID without laparoscopic confirmation, we should use all relevant information obtained from the patient to weigh for and against the diagnosis (Table 4.2). Hager and coworkers[37] suggested certain clinical criteria for a diagnosis of acute PID. For the sake of uniformity, it was fortunate that many investigators used these criteria in PID studies. However, the criteria have never been validated in a laparoscopic study, and are now regarded as obsolete.[3] In a single case of pelvic pain, whichever clinical criteria are used, it is important to keep in mind that the diagnosis might be wrong. One should therefore reevaluate the patient after a few days and revise the diagnosis if deemed appropriate.

TABLE 4.2. Information that points towards or against a diagnosis of acute PID in women with pelvic pain.

PID more likely	Information	PID less likely
Yes	New sexual partner	No
Yes	History of IUD	No
Yes	Recently introduced IUD	No
Gradual	Pain debut	Sudden
<3 weeks	Pain duration	>3 weeks
Constant	Pain character	Intermittent
Bilateral	Pain localization	Unilateral
Heavy	Last menstruation	Light or late
No	Oral contraceptive use	Yes
No	Tubal ligation	Yes
Negative	Pregnancy test	Positive
>15 mm/h	ESR	<15 mm/h
>6 mg/L	CRP	<6 mg/L
Positive	Chlamydial or gonococcal culture	Negative
Fluid filled, thickened walls	Fallopian tubes on ultrasonography	Not seen

Silent Pelvic Inflammatory Disease

"Silent" PID is a term used for the infection causing the tubal scarring often found in infertile women with no history of PID. A high percentage of these women have serum antibodies to *C. trachomatis*.[20,38] In retrospect, these women have had PID. We do not know, however, whether the infection was asymptomatic (silent), disregarded by the patient and therefore never identified, or misdiagnosed by the physician and therefore never treated. However, in a recent study, infertile women were asked whether they had sought medical advice for any lower abdominal pain.[39] Among 36 women with pelvic adhesions and/or distal tubal occlusion, only 4 had no history of abdominal pain and no evidence of endometriosis. This study suggests that silent PID might not be as common as previously thought. The clinical manifestations, if any, of silent PID are unknown, Therefore, we cannot make the diagnosis of silent PID in the acute stage. Possibly, menorrhagia and mucopurulent cervicitis are manifestations of silent PID in some women.[40] For example, among women not using oral contraceptives, menorrhagia correlates with chlamydial and gonococcal infection (Wølner-Hanssen and coworkers, unpublished data). About one-half of women with mucopurulent cervicitis have histopathological evidence of endometritis.[41] However, the status of the fallopian tubes in women with mucopurulent cervicitis or menorrhagia is unknown.

Patients with PID who delay medical care, increase the risk of infertility and ectopic pregnancy.[42] Patients not seeking care at all will probably have even higher risk of infertility. An unknown part of infertile women diagnosed as having had silent PID certainly belong to the latter. Therefore, we need to put more efforts in educating young women about the manifestations of PID.

Summary

Acute PID produces nonspecific and variable signs and symptoms. The organs of most interest, the fallopian tubes, are not immediately visible and only indirectly palpable. No good algorithm for the clinical diagnosis of PID is available. Recent developments in the area of PID diagnostics include the new, extremely sensitive pregnancy tests, endometrial biopsy, rapid tests for *C. trachomatis*, and ultrasonography. None of these developments can replace laparoscopy as the gold standard for PID diagnostics, however. In the future, then, routine health care will continue having to deal with the uncertainties of PID diagnostics.

References

1. Bongard F, Landers D, Lewis F. Differential diagnosis of appendicitis and pelvic inflammatory disease. *Am J Surg* 1985;**150**:90–96.

2. Weström L. *Diagnosis, Aetiology, and Prognosis of Acute Salpingitis*, thesis. Studentlitteratur, Lund, Sweden, 1976.
3. Kahn JG, Walker CK, Washington E, et al. Diagnosing pelvic inflammatory disease. A comprehensive analysis and considerations for developing a new model. *JAMA* 1991;**266**:2594–2604.
4. Wølner-Hanssen P, Mårdh P-A, Svensson L, et al. Laparoscopy in women with chlamydial infection and pelvic pain: A comparison of patients with and without salpingitis. *Obstet Gynecol* 1983;**61**:299–303.
5. Hadgu A, Weström L, Brooks CA, et al. Predicting pelvic inflammatory disease: A multivariate analysis. *Am J Obstet Gynecol* 1986;**155**:954–960.
6. Tavelli BG, Judson FN. Comparison of the clinical and epidemiologic characteristics of gonococcal and nongonococcal pelvic inflammatory disease seen in a clinic for sexually transmitted diseases, 1978–1979. *Sex Transm Dis* 1986;**13**: 119–122.
7. Wølner-Hanssen P, Eschenbach DA, Paavonen J, et al. Decreased risk of chlamydial pelvic inflammatory disease associated with oral contraceptive use. *JAMA* 1990;**263**:54–59.
8. Wølner-Hanssen P, Svensson L, Mårdh P-A, Weström L. Laparoscopic findings and contraceptive use in women with signs and symptoms suggestive of acute salpingitis. *Obstet Gynecol* 1985;**66**:233–238.
9. Svensson L, Weström L, Mårdh P-A. Contraceptives and acute salpingitis. *JAMA* 1984;**251**:2553–2555.
10. Wølner-Hanssen P. Oral contraceptive use modifies the manifestations of pelvic inflammatory disease. *Br J Obstet Gynecol* 1986;**93**:619–624.
11. Washington AE, Gove S, Schachter J, Sweet RL. Oral contraceptives, *Chlamydia trachomatis* infection, and pelvic inflammatory disease: A word of caution about protection. *JAMA* 1985;**253**:2246–2250.
12. Hajj SN. Does sterilization prevent pelvic infection? *J Reprod Med* 1978;**20**:289.
13. Fletcher V Jr. Proximal stump salpingitis. *Am J Obstet Gynecol* 1986;**155**: 496–500.
14. Blanchard AC, Pastorek JG, Weeks T. Pelvic inflammatory disease during pregnancy. *South Med J* 1987;**80**:1363–1365.
15. Lehtinen M, Laine S, Heinonen PK, et al. Serum C-reactive protein determination in acute pelvic inflammatory disease. *Am J Obstet Gynecol* 1986;**154**: 158–159.
16. Hemilä M, Henriksson L, Ylikorkala O. Serum CRP in the diagnosis and treatment of pelvic inflammatory disease. *Arch Gynecol Obstet* 1987;**241**: 177–182.
17. Schmidt-Rhode P, Schulz K-D, Sturm G, et al. C-reactive protein is a marker for the diagnosis of adnexitis. *Int J Obstet Gynecol* 1990;**32**:133–139.
18. Jacobson L, Weström L. Objectivized diagnosis of pelvic inflammatory disease. *Am J Obstet Gynecol* 1969;**105**:1088–1098.
19. Treharne J, Ripa KT, Mårdh P-A, et al. Antibodies to *Chlamydia trachomatis* in acute salpingitis. *Br J Vener Dis* 1979;**55**:26–29.
20. Moore DE, Spadoni LR, Foy HM, et al. Increased frequency of serum antibodies to *Chlamydia trachomatis* in infertility due to distal tubal disease. Lancet 1982;**ii**:574–577.
21. Osborne NG, Hecht Y, Gorsline J, et al. A comparison of culture, direct fluorescent antibody test, and a quantitative indirect immunoperoxidase assay

for detection of *Chlamydia trachomatis* in pregnant women. *Obstet Gynecol* 1988;**71**:412–415.

22. Brunham RC, Paavonen J, Stevens C, et al. Mucopurulent cervicitis: The ignored counterpart in women of urethritis in men. *N Engl J Med* 1984;**311**:1–6.

23. Willmott FE. Mucopurulent cervicitis: A clinical entity? *Genitourin Med* 1988;**64**:169–171.

24. Moscicki B, Shafer M-A, Millstein SG, et al. The use and limitations of endocervical Gram stains and mucopurulent cervicitis as predictors for *Chlamydia trachomatis* in female adolescents. *Am J Obstet Gynecol* 1987;**157**:65–71.

25. Larsson P-G, Platz-Christensen JJ. Bacterial vaginosis and the vaginal leucocyte/epithelial cell ratio in women attending an outpatient gynaecology clinic. *Eur J Obstet Gynecol Reprod Biol* 1991;**38**:39–41.

26. Paavonen J, Aine R, Teisala K, et al. Comparison of endometrial biopsy and peritoneal fluid cytologic testing with laparoscopy in the diagnosis of acute pelvic inflammatory disease. *Am J Obstet Gynecol* 1985;**151**:645–650.

27. Sweet RL, Mills J, Hadley KW, et al. Use of laparoscopy to determine the microbiologic etiology of acute salpingitis. *Am J Obstet Gynecol* 1979;**134**:68–74.

28. Weström L. Effect of acute pelvic inflammatory disease on fertility. *Am J Obstet Gynecol* 1975;**121**:707–713.

29. Miettinen AK, Heinonnen PK, Laippala P, Paavonen J. Test performance of erythrocyte sedimentation rate and C-reactive protein in assessing the severity of acute pelvic inflammatory disease. *Am J Obstet Gynecol* 1993;**169**:1143–1149.

30. Stacey C, Munday P, Thomas B, et al. *Chlamydia trachomatis* in the fallopian tubes of women without laparoscopic evidence of salpingitis. *Lancet* 1990;**ii**:960–963.

31. Sellors J, Mahony J, Goldsmith C, et al. The accuracy of clinical findings and laparoscopy in pelvic inflammatory disease. *Am J Obstet Gynecol* 1991;**164**:113–120.

32. Kiviat N, Wølner-Hanssen P, Eschenbach D, et al. Endometrial histopathology in patients with culture-proven upper genital tract infection and laparoscopically diagnosed acute salpingitis. *Am J Surg Pathol* 1990;**14(2)**:167–175.

33. Cacciatore B, Leminen A, Ingman-Friberg S, et al. Transvaginal sonographic findings in ambulatory patients with suspected pelvic inflammatory disease. *Obstet Gynecol* 1992;**80**:912–916.

34. Patten RM, Vincent LM, Wølner-Hanssen P, et al. Pelvic inflammatory disease: Endovaginal sonography with laparoscopic correlation. *J Ultrasound Med* 1990;**9**:681–689.

35. Puylaert JBCM, Rutgers PH, Lalisang RI, et al. A prospecitve study of ultrasonography in the diagnosis of appendicitis. *N Engl J Med* 1987;**317**:666–669.

36. Weström L. Clinical manifestations and diagnosis of pelvic inflammatory disease. *J Reprod Med* 1983;**28**(suppl):703–708.

37. Hager WD, Eschenbach DA, Spence MR, Sweet RL. Criteria for diagnosis and grading of salpingitis. *Obstet Gynecol* 1983;**61**:113–114.

38. Punnonen R, Terho P, Nikkanen V, et al. Chlamydial serology in infertile women by immunofluorescence. *Fertil Steril* 1979;**31**:656–659.

39. Wølner-Hanssen P. Silent pelvic inflammatory disease: Is it overstated? *Obstet Gynecol* 1995;**86**:321–325.

40. Wølner-Hanssen P, Kiviat NK, Holmes KK. Atypical pelvic inflammatory disease: Subacute, chronic, or subclinical upper genital tract infection in women. In Holmes KK, Mårdh P-A, Sparling PF, Wiesner PJ (eds): *Sexually Transmitted Diseases*. 2nd ed. New York, McGraw-Hill Book Company, 1989, pp 615–620.
41. Paavonen J, Kiviat N, Brunham R, et al. Prevalence and manifestations of endometritis among women with cervicitis. *Am J Obstet Gynecol* 1985;**152**: 280–286.
42. Hillis SD, Joesoef R, Marchbanks PA, et al. Delayed care of pelvic inflammatory disease as a risk factor for impaired fertility. *Am J Obstet Gynecol* 1993;**168**:1503–1509.

5
Treatment of Acute Pelvic Inflammatory Disease

RICHARD L. SWEET

The optimum strategy for minimizing the sequelae is prevention of pelvic inflammatory disease (PID) by preventing lower genital tract infections such as cervicitis with *Neisseria gonorrhoeae* or *Chlamydia trachomatis* and bacterial vaginosis (BV) (i.e., primary prevention).[1] A secondary approach, when primary prevention fails, relies on early detection and prompt treatment of lower genital tract infections. Unfortunately accomplishing either of these two strategies requires effective sexually transmitted disease (STD) control programs, which to date are sorely lacking in the United States. Thus, in the United States prevention of these sequelae relies on prompt diagnosis and treatment of acute PID. This so-called tertiary prevention approach is further complicated by the wide spectrum of clinical presentation of PID, ranging from asymptomatic ("silent") to minimally symptomatic ("atypical" or "unrecognized") to clinical PID ("typical"). Whether patients are truly asymptomatic or unrecognized because they present with minimal or atypical signs and symptoms of PID has been uncertain. Recently, Wølner-Hanssen[2] provided data demonstrating that patients listed as having silent PID truly did have symptoms suggestive of PID when questioned extensively.

The main goals in the treatment of acute PID are to resolve the acute inflammatory process, preserve fertility, prevent ectopic pregnancy, and reduce the likelihood of chronic pelvic pain. A delay in the initiation of therapy is hazardous; treatment early in the course of acute PID has been shown to be beneficial in the preservation of tubal patency.[3] Data obtained from an animal model of chlamydial PID also suggest that early treatment may prevent infertility.[4,5]

Older treatment strategies were based on single-agent narrow-spectrum antimicrobials with eradication of *N. gonorrhoeae* as their main objective. The high failure rates associated with these regimens can be explained easily by their failure to eradicate mixed aerobic-anaerobic bacteria and *C. trachomatis*, which have been shown to play major roles in the pathogenesis of most cases of acute PID. In recognition of the polymicrobial etiology of acute PID, recent guidelines established by The Centers for Disease Control (CDC) have recommended specific broad-spectrum antibiotic regimens.[6] Inpatient and ambulatory treatment recommendations provide coverage against *N. gonorrhoeae*, *C. trachomatis*, and anaerobes and facultative aerobic organisms. There are a myriad of antibiotics commonly used to treat PID. The majority of these are extensions of the two CDC recommended regimens. The clinician may be confused by the extensive list of single agents and combinations available to them. Furthermore, the literature on antibiotic efficacy in treating PID may be complicated and confusing. In this chapter, commonly used antimicrobial regimens for treating PID will be examined for hospitalized and ambulatory management.

Successful treatment of acute PID has historically been gauged by clinical and/or microbiological evidence of cure. In published studies, these endpoints have included resolution of symptoms and abnormal physical findings, and eradication of microbial pathogens. Virtually all published studies on antibiotic-efficacy for the treatment of PID have relied on these endpoints. While these short-term objectives are crucial, prevention of later consequences, specifically tubal damage, are equally important long-term objectives in the management of acute PID. Unfortunately, there is a paucity of data on these long-term outcomes, and such conclusions of antimicrobial efficacy must be based on the achievement of the above-mentioned short-term goals. Future studies on the efficacy of different treatment regimens of PID in the prevention of long-term sequelae will play an important role in optimizing PID treatment.

The majority of women with acute PID are treated in ambulatory settings. In the 1980s, hospitalization rates for acute PID steadily declined, decreasing 36% over a 10-year period from 1979 to 1988.[1] Some experts strongly believe in aggressive in-patient management of all patients with PID. The main theoretical impetus for this approach is that parenteral treatment delivers high doses of antibiotics, yielding the highest tissue levels and thereby improved efficacy. There are additional important factors favoring hospitalization. Treatment compliance is virtually assured in the controlled environment of the hospital. Unfortunately, lack of compliance is a major drawback in outpatient treatment of PID. The issue is especially relevant for PID, as the highest risk individuals for this infection, namely adolescents, are notoriously noncompliant with all medical treatments. Treatment failures are more apt to the detected earlier in those women who are hospitalized, facilitating a potentially beneficial change in management. Managing these patients in a hospitalized setting further enables daily aggressive and comprehensive education programs, such as prevention counseling. Opportunity for effective counseling may be limited in an ambulatory setting.

Etiology and Pathogenesis

The etiology of PID is thought to be polymicrobic in nature and thus multiple organisms have been implicated as etiological agents in the disease.[7–9] *Neisseria gonorrhoeae*, *C. trachomatis*, and a wide variety of anaerobic and aerobic bacteria are recognized as playing an etiological role in PID. The most common anaerobic bacteria involved are *Prevotella* (previously *Bacteroides* spp), especially *P. bivia*, and *Peptostreptococcus* spp. The most common facultative bacteria are *Gardnerella vaginalis*, *Streptococcus* species, *Escherichia coli*, and *Haemophilius influenzae*. Recently the syndrome BV has demonstrated to be an antecedent lower genital tract infection that leads to acute PID.[8,10–12] It has also been suggested that mycoplasmas play a role in PID but their role is controversial.[13] Reports by Rice and Schachter,[14] and Jossens et al.[15] demonstrated that most cases of PID are associated with *N. gonorrhoeae* and/or *C. trachomatis*. Jossens et al. demonstrated, in a large series ($n = 589$) of hospitalized cases with acute PID, *N. gonorrhoeae* and/or *C. trachomatis* were present in 65% of the cases. In 30% of the cases only anaerobic and/or facultative bacteria were isolated. While, in addition, anaerobic and/or facultative organisms were frequently (nearly 50%) recovered from the upper genital tract of patients demonstrated to have either *N. gonorrhoeae* or *C. trachomatis*. Rice and Schachter[14] have also noted that 25% to 50% of PID cases do not have detectable chlamydial or gonococcal infection, but only have anaerobic and facultative bacteria isolated from the upper genital tract.

Pelvic inflammatory disease results from direct canalicular spread of microorganisms from the lower genital tract to the endometrial cavity and fallopian tube.[14] It is generally believed that 10% to 15% of women with cervicitis due to *N. gonorrhoeae* or *C. trachomatis* will go on to develop PID.[16] However, reports as high as 40% of women treated for gonococcal or chlamydial cervicitis develop clinical symptoms suggestive of PID.[17,18] Even higher percentages of ascending infection are present if endometrial biopsies are used to diagnose histological endometritis.[1] Similarly, patients with BV also have been shown to have a high incidence of histological endometritis unrelated to *C. trachomatis* or *N. gonorrhoeae*.[11] The CDC has suggested that certain factors may contribute to the ascent of microorganisms to the upper genital tract.[1] These include: (1) uterine instrumentation (such as insertion of an intrauterine device [IUD]), which can facilitate a port of ascent of vaginal and cervical bacteria; (2) hormonal changes during menses as well as menstruation itself lead to cervical alterations that may result in the loss of a mechanical barrier preventing ascent; (3) the bacteriostatic effect of cervical mucous is low at the onset of menses; (4) retrograde menstruation may favor ascent to the tubes and peritoneum; and (5) individual organisms may have potential virulence factors associated with the pathogenesis of acute chlamydial and gonococcal PID.[1]

While the major therapeutic goal in the treatment of acute PID is prevention of infertility, ectopic pregnancy and the chronic residua of infection, the overwhelming majority of data on the treatment of acute PID focus on the short-term outcomes of initial clinical response and microbiological eradication. Literature from the preantibiotic era demonstrates that many cases of acute PID managed with only conservative, supportive therapy resolve spontaneously and without sequelae.[19–21] As reported by Curtis,[20,22] 85% of patients with acute PID improved without surgery, whereas the remaining 15% had prolonged, progressive symptoms that culminated in surgical intervention. Similarly, Holtz,[19] in a review of 1,262 patients, demonstrated excellent results with conservative therapy; there was a 9% incidence of persistent, severe symptoms, a 6% incidence of fever present for longer than 2 months and 1.3% incidence of mortality. Early studies from Scandinavia in the late 1950s and early 1960s suggested that antibiotics had improved the prognosis for the long-term outcome of acute PID. In these reports mortality had been virtually eliminated; the frequency of ruptured tubo-ovarian abscesses and persistent abscesses requiring surgery had decreased; and the fertility rates had notably improved.[23–25] The Holtz study,[19] from the preantibiotic era, demonstrated nearly a 23% pregnancy rate in patients with gonococcal PID. The early Scandinavian studies reported that the use of antibiotics in the treatment of gonococcal PID resulted in crude pregnancy rates ranging from 39% to 51%.[19–23] In these studies, when the patients who were voluntary infertile or in whom surgical intervention had been necessary were excluded, the corrected pregnancy rates ranged from 67% to 84%.[19–23] Among the women with nongonococcal PID, antibiotic treatment resulted in crude pregnancy rates ranging from 25% to 44% with corrected pregnancy rates ranging from 60% to 81%.[3,19,25]

In a recent review Weström and Berger[26] summarized the prospective studies that assessed fertility following episodes of acute PID; they compared studies prior to and after the introduction of antibiotic therapy for the treatment of acute PID. These studies (Table 5.1) demonstrated that fertility generally improved following the introduction of antibiotic therapy. In these reports the mean pregnancy rate in women attempting pregnancy was 27.9% in the preantibiotic era versus 73.1% following the advent of antibiotic treatment. Among the patients in the preantibiotic era, pregnancy rates ranged from 24% to 43%, while after antibiotic therapy the range was 24 to 81%.[3,19,23,27–29,30–32] More recently, Safrin et al.[33] reported pregnancy rates that were much less optimistic with an infertility rate of 40%. Thus, similar to the study by Brunham et al.[34] with an infertility rate of 30%, pregnancy rates in North America have been associated with much poorer prognosis than those reported from Scandinavian studies.

While initial evaluation suggests that antimicrobial therapy has resulted in improved prognosis for fertility following acute PID, the results are far from satisfactory. Higher pregnancy rates associated with antibiotic therapy are corrected rates that have excluded patients for whom the infection

TABLE 5.1. Follow-up studies of fertility in women with PID in the preantibiotic and postantibiotic eras.

Study	Women with follow-up (N)	Antibiotic therapy	Pregnancy rates Unadjusted* (%)	Adjusted[†] (%)
Holtz[19] (1930)	804	No	17	25
Hubscher[27] (1993)	133	No	23	—
Haffner[28] (1939)	169	No	27	43
Hedberg and Spetz[29] (1958)	138	Yes	30	63
Viberg[3] (1964)	54	Yes	23	24
	53	No	22	24
Falk[23] (1965)	281	Yes	47	81
Weström[36] (1975)	Yes	Yes	63	79
Weström[31] (1982)	900	Yes	65	80
Brunham[34] (1988)	23	Yes	22	50
Safrin[33] (1992)	140	Yes	—	60

*Those with follow-up.
[†] Patients followed-up and exposed to chance of pregnancy.

resulted in surgical intervention that precluded future fertility. Exclusion of these patients may prevent an accurate assessment of the true prognosis for fertility, as the rates in the uncorrected groups were similar. Moreover, recent studies in North America,[33,34] using adjusted rates of pregnancy, have demonstrated a much poorer prognosis than the earlier Scandinavian reports.[35,36] Weström,[36] in a classic, long-term longitudinal study of women with laparoscopy-confirmed salpingitis, reported that despite antibiotic therapy, patients with at least one episode of acute PID had a 21% rate of involuntary infertility compared with a rate of 3% in the control population. In addition, despite antibiotic therapy, a sixfold increase in the incidence of ectopic pregnancies was noted in these salpingitis patients. In this study, Weström also noted that the prognosis for infertility was directly related to the number of episodes of salpingitis. With a single episode, the risk of infertility was approximately 11%, rising to 34% with two episodes, and to 54% following three or more episodes of acute salpingitis. In this large cohort, Weström and coworkers[37] reported that in a group of 604 laparoscopy confirmed cases of first episode acute PID, the infertility rate on long-term follow-up ranged from 10% to 13% regardless of the type of antibiotic regimen that had been utilized. However, none of the regimens used (penicillin plus streptomycin, ampicillin alone, ampicillin and doxycycline, and doxycycline alone) provided adequate coverage for the three major etiological groups of organisms involved in polymicrobic PID: N. gonorrhoeae, C. trachomatis, and anaerobic/aerobic bacteria. More recently Weström updated this series to a total of 1,844 cases of acute PID.[35] The rate of tubal factor infertility rose from 8.0% with one episode to

19.5% with two episodes and 40% with three or more episodes. Overall the infertility rate was 10.8%.[35]

In the Weström laparoscopy studies,[36] patients with gonococcal salpingitis were noted to have a better prognosis for future fertility than those with nongonococcal disease. This result is probably due to several factors: (1) patients with gonococcal disease present with a classically described complex of high fever, leukocytosis and purulent discharge from the cervix, in addition to the findings of cervical motion tenderness and adnexal tenderness; (2) physicians relying on these classic signs and symptoms of acute PID diagnose gonococcal disease more often and treat it earlier than nongonococcal disease; (3) patients with gonococcal disease tend to meet the criteria utilized for hospital admission and thus are admitted early in their disease course and treated with intravenous antibiotics that include adequate coverage against *N. gonorrhoeae*; (4) failure to recognize the importance of *C. trachomatis* as an etiological agent in acute PID and the role it plays in adverse outcomes; and (5) failure to include coverage against anaerobic bacteria. As a result of these factors, it should not be a surprise to find that patients with gonococcal disease who are diagnosed and treated appropriately have a better prognosis for fertility. Recently Brunham et al.[32] have confirmed this finding in a Canadian study that prospectively assessed post-PID fertility. In this study the authors reported that all patients with gonococcal PID who attempted to conceive did so successfully. On the other hand, those patients with nongonococcal disease who had presented with milder symptoms often had a poorer prognosis for future fertility. In particular, Brunham et al. noted that *C. trachomatis* and anaerobic bacteria associated with pyosalpinges or tubo-ovarian abscesses were associated with poor prognosis for future fertility. At this time it is not clear whether any particular nongonococcal pathogen such as *C. trachomatis*, anaerobic bacteria, or mycoplasmas are associated with a worse prognosis for future fertility. Initially, Weström et al. suggested that those patients with chlamydial salpingitis, as determined by either the presence of serological confirmation of *C. trachomatis* with significant antibody titer rises or by recovery of the organism from the fallopian tube, were more likely to have severe inflammatory involvement of the fallopian tube at laparoscopy and the worst prognosis for future fertility.[30,36] However, more recently, this group, utilizing only cervical cultures, noted that there was no difference in the involuntary infertility rate among women with chlamydial salpingitis, gonococcal salpingitis, chlamydial and gonococcal salpingitis, or nongonococcal, nonchlamydial salpingitis.[38] In this study, the rates of infertility were 22.7%, 23.5%, 20%, and 22%, respectively.[38] Clearly, as discussed in Chapter 11 on the sequelae of acute PID, the presence of IgG antichlamydial antibody has been associated with tubal factor infertility and ectopic pregnancies.

Early diagnosis and treatment of PID are critical to the preservation of future fertility. Several studies have demonstrated that the ability of antimicrobial therapy to prevent infertility is dependent upon the interval between the onset of symptoms and the institution of treatment.[3,23,24] In these studies, which utilized hysterosalpingogram and/or laparoscopy, women who had been treated early in the course of their acute episode of PID had tubal patency present in large numbers. Viberg[3] reported that none of the patients treated within 2 days of the onset of symptoms was involuntary infertile and that all had patent fallopian tubes on hysterosalpingogram. However, if treatment had been instituted on day 7 or later, only 70% of the patients were shown to have tubal patency with hysterosalpingogram. More recently, Hillis et al.,[39] in a study utilizing the Weström database, demonstrated that women who had been treated after 3 or more days of symptoms had a significantly greater infertility rate than those who had been treated after less than 3 days of symptomatology (19.7% vs. 8.3%).[39] A similar short window of opportunity within 5 to 6 days of disease onset has been demonstrated in animal model studies of acute chlamydial PID as well.[4,5]

In addition to the need for antibiotic therapy to be instituted early in the disease process for it to be effective, an antibiotic regimen must be utilized that takes into account the polymicrobial nature of acute PID. The major pathogens associated with PID include *C. trachomatis, N. gonorrhoeae, Prevotella* species, *Peptostreptococcus* species, and aerobic bacteria such as *Gardnerella vaginalis, E. coli, facultative streptococci*, and *Haemophilus influenzae*. Whether it is necessary to cover all these organisms is not proven. However, Brunham et al.[34] have reported that PID associated with *C. trachomatis* and anaerobic bacteria were associated with the worst prognosis for post-PID infertility.

The issue of outpatient treatment versus inpatient treatment for PID has been controversial. Unfortunately, there are no data available that prospectively evaluate the need for hospital versus ambulatory management of acute PID. Nor is data available as to the efficacy of oral antibiotics versus parenteral antibiotics. Due, in large part, to economic and logistic reasons, especially in the era of managed care, less than 20% to 25% of patients with acute PID are hospitalized in the United States. The CDC has published recommended treatment regimens for acute PID. The most current recommendations are provided in Tables 5.2 and 5.3.[1] These regimens are based on the premise that it is necessary to cover all the major etiological agents involved in acute PID, including *N. gonorrhoeae, C. trachomatis*, anaerobic bacteria such as *Prevotella* species and *Peptostreptococcus* species and gram-negative aerobes such as *E. coli, Gardnerella vaginalis*, and *Haemophilus influenzae*.

Once a diagnosis of acute PID has been made, a decision must be made as to whether to hospitalize or treat on an ambulatory basis. There currently is no satisfactory answer to this dilemma and the controversy between ambulatory and hospital management is still present. Indications for hospitalization among patients with acute PID have been suggested. Those that

TABLE 5.2. Centers for Disease Control recommended treatment schedules for ambulatory management of acute pelvic inflammatory disease—1993.

Regimen	Treatment
A	Cefoxitin 2 g i.m. plus probenecid 1 g p.o. in a single dose concurrently, or ceftrixaone 250 mg i.m. or other parenteral third-generation cephalosporin (e.g., ceftizoxime or cefoxtaxime)
	PLUS
	Doxycycline 100 mg p.o. 2 times a day for 14 days
B	Ofloxacin 400 mg p.o. 2 times a day for 14 days
	PLUS
	Either clindamycin 450 mg p.o. 4 times a day, or metronidazole 500 mg p.o. 2 times a day for 14 days

Source: MMWR 1993;**42**:75–81.

we use are listed in Table 5.4. The question of whether all patients should be treated on a hospitalized basis or in a home parenteral therapy program with combination parenteral therapy remains to be determined. Such a decision will require prospective randomized trials involving ambulatory and hospitalized treatment regimens. In addition, such studies must not only assess short-term results, such as clinical response and microbiological eradication, but must assess long-term outcome, such as infertility and ectopic pregnancy rates. It is of great importance that those patients who

TABLE 5.3. Centers for Disease Control recommended treatment schedules for acute pelvic inflammatory disease—1993.

Inpatient treatment	
1.	Cefoxitin 2 g i.v. every 6 h
	OR
	Cefotetan* 2 g i.v. every 12 h
	PLUS
	Doxycycline 100 mg every 12 h p.o. or i.v.
	(Regimen given for at least 48 h after patient clinically improves. After discharge from hospital, continue doxycycline 100 mg p.o. twice a day for a total of 14 days)
2.	Clindamycin 900 mg i.v. every 8 h
	PLUS
	Gentamicin loading dose i.v. or i.m. (2 mg/kg) followed by maintenance dose (1.5 mg/kg) every 8 h
	(Regimen given for at least 48 h after the patient improves. After discharge from the hospital, continue doxycycline 100 mg p.o. twice a day for 14 days total or clindamycin 450 mg p.o. 5 times daily for 10–14 days)

* Other cephalosporins such as ceftizoxime, cefotaxime, and ceftriaxone that provide adequate gonococcal, other facultative gram-negative aerobic, and anaerobic coverage may be used in appropriate doses.
Source: MMWR 1993;**42**:75–81.

TABLE 5.4. Criteria for hospitalization of patients with acute pelvic inflammatory disease.

1.	All acute pelvic inflammatory disease cases?
2.	Suspected pelvic or tubo-ovarian abscess
3.	Pregnancy
4.	Temperature $> 38°C$
5.	Uncertain diagnosis
6.	Nausea and vomiting precluding oral medications
7.	Upper peritoneal signs
8.	Failure to respond to oral antibiotics within 48 h
9.	Adolescents

have not responded promptly to ambulatory therapy be reevaluated and hospitalized for parenteral therapy. We believe that the critical evaluation point is 48 h after commencement of ambulatory therapy. We feel strongly also that those women with suspected tubo-ovarian abscesses require hospitalization for parenteral therapy and close monitoring. Many authorities recommend that adolescents with acute PID be hospitalized. This recommendation is based on the high-noncompliance rate among the adolescent population with the use of multiple doses of antimicrobial therapy. Katz and coworkers[40] have reported that only 63% of adolescent patients with chlamydial infection completed a standard 7-day regimen of tetracycline. The factors leading to failure to comply with the standard regimen include lack of patients education or perception regarding therapeutic value, complex dosing regimens, inconvenient administration route, high-cost medications, and adverse reactions, especially gastrointestinal side effects.[40]

The CDC recommendations have relied on using combinations of agents to cover the multitude of microorganisms involved in the polymicrobial etiology of acute PID. In fact, the CDC recommends that single-agent therapy is not appropriate for the management of acute PID. With the regimens for hospitalized care of PID (Table 5.3), the cefoxitin plus doxycycline regimen appears to provide coverage against all the major pathogen groups. While doxycycline is active against *C. trachomatis*, cefoxitin provides excellent coverage against *N. gonorrhoeae* (including most penicillinase-producing strains), gram-positive aerobes (especially *Streptococci*), gram-negative aerobes such as *E. coli*, and penicillin-sensitive and nonpenicillin-sensitive anaerobic bacteria, including the *Prevotella* species. Cefotetan is an excellent alternative to cefoxitin with the added advantage of twice-a-day dosing versus four-times-a-day dosing with cefoxitin. Sweet et al.[41] prospectively compared cefoxitin plus doxycycline with cefotetan plus doxycycline for the treatment of acute PID and noted equal and excellent initial clinical efficacy in microbiological eradication with both regimens. The clinical cure rates were 94% in the cefotetan group and 92% with the cefoxitin regimen. At 1 week and 3 weeks post-treatment, all instances of *N. gonorrhoeae* and *C. trachomatis* had been eradicated. These regimens were also effective in eradicating anaerobic and aerobe pathogens from the endometrial cavity in the post-treatment analysis.

While the clindamycin plus gentamicin regimen provides excellent coverage against anaerobic bacteria, gram-negative aerobes and gram-positive aerobes, concern has been raised over its activity against *C. trachomatis* and *N. gonorrhoeae*. While *in vitro* studies demonstrated that clindamycin is effective against maximally 90% of *C. trachomatis* strains,[42] its efficacy in clinical cases of chlamydial PID has been recently demonstrated. Wasserheit et al.[43] reported that clindamycin effectively eradicated *C. trachomatis* in 100% of cases of chlamydial salpingitis. Similarly, Sweet et al.[44] confirmed the clinical efficacy of clindamycin against *C. trachomatis* in patients with acute PID. Neither clindamycin nor aminoglycosides are the agent of choice against *N. gonorrhoeae* but they are both effective against nonpenicillinase-producing strains.[45] Although discussed in Chapter 6 on tubo-ovarian abscesses, cefoxitin plus doxycycline and clindamycin plus gentamicin regimens provide excellent activity in the face of tubo-ovarian abscesses with clinical cure rates of antibiotic therapy alone in the area of 75%.[46] Thus, both of these regimens are safe to utilize when it is unclear whether an abscess is present or not.

The 1993 CDC guidelines for the antimicrobial therapy of PID on an ambulatory basis are provided in Table 5.2. With regimen A the cefoxitin plus doxycycline is similar to that used for hospitalized treatment except the cefoxitin is provided as a single dose. This has led to concern that anaerobic coverage is not sufficient in the ambulatory regimen. If ceftrixaone is used as the cephalosporin in regimen A it provides poor anaerobic coverage and again for only a single dose. The same is true for other parenteral third-generation cephalosporins. The inclusion of ofloxacin plus either clindamycin or metronidazole in the 1993 guidelines was an attempt to answer the concern over anaerobic coverage in the ambulatory regimens.[1] In this regimen, ofloxacin covers *N. gonorrhoeae* and *C. trachomatis*, while clindamycin or metronidazole provide coverage for anaerobic bacteria including *Prevotella* species and *Peptostreptococci*. In addition, ofloxacin is active against gram-negative enterics such as *E. coli* and clindamycin is active against aerobic streptococci.

Few microbiologically controlled prospective randomized clinical trials comparing the various antibiotic regimens for the treatment of acute PID have been reported. Recently Walker et al.[47] performed a meta-analysis of antibiotic regimen efficacy for the treatment of acute PID.[47] In this meta-analysis 34 treatment studies published between 1966 and 1992 were identified. Of these, 21 met the criteria for inclusion having used an appropriate system for making the diagnosis of PID a standardized assessment of clinical outcome and entry and follow-up evaluation for cervical infection with *N. gonorrhoeae* and *C. trachomatis*. Tables 5.5 and 5.6 summarize the pooled clinical cure rates in these studies with clinical cure rates ranging

TABLE 5.5. Reported pooled cure rates in treatment of acute PID for antibiotic regimens with more than one study included in the meta-analysis by Walker et al.[47]

Drug regimen	No. of studies	No. of patients	Clinical cure rate (%)	Microbiological cure rate* (%)
Inpatient				
Clindamycin + aminoglycoside	10	372	92	97
Cefoxitin + doxycycline	7	338	93	98
Cefotetan + doxycycline	2	86	94	100
Ciprofloxacin	4	90	94	96[†]
Metronidazole + doxycycline	2	36	75	71
Outpatient				
Cefoxitin + doxycycline	2	59	95	91

*Microbiological cure based on eradication of N. gonorrhoeae and C. trachomatis.
[†]High rate of persistent anaerobic bacteria noted.

from 75% to 94%. The pooled microbiological cure rates ranged from 77% to 100%. With the exception of the metronidazole plus doxycycline regimen, these antimicrobial regimens appear to have excellent short-term clinical and microbiological efficacy. The antimicrobial spectrum of activity and costs of these regimens are provided in Table 5.7. Unfortunately, these studies do not address the effect of therapy on long-term outcomes such as infertility, ectopic pregnancies, and recurrent PID. Such studies are clearly necessary to determine whether all potential pathogens must be covered by antimicrobial therapy. In addition, no well-controlled studies to date have compared short- or long-term outcomes of outpatient versus inpatient therapy. At the present time, to ensure the best possible prognosis for future fertility and to prevent other serious long-term sequelae, vigorous inpatient parenteral therapy coupled with careful outpatient follow-up is the optimum approach. However, because of the economic realities of managed care, outpatient therapy has been increasingly utilized.

Dodson[48] also recently reported a statisticial analysis of 58 studies that involved 101 clinical trials with over 4,000 patients for the antibiotic treat-. ment of acute PID. In particular, Dodson compared the results of 12

TABLE 5.6. Reported cure rates in treatment of acute PID for antibiotic regimens with only single study in the meta-analysis by Walker et al.[47]

Drug Regimen	No. of patients	Clinical cure rate (%)	Microbiological cure rate* (%)
Inpatient			
Ceftizoxime + tetracycline	18	88	100
Cefotaxime + tetracycline	19	94	100
Sulbactam-ampicillin + doxycycline	37	95	100
Outpatient			
Amoxicillin-clavulanic acid	35	100	100
Ofloxacin	37	95	100

*Eradication of N. gonorrhoeae and C. trachomatis.

TABLE 5.7. Antimicrobial activity of regimens included in the meta-analysis.*

Drug regimen	Cost ($)/day†	N. gonorrhoeae Non-PP	N. gonorrhoeae PP	C. trachomatis	Anaerobic bacteria Non-PP	Anaerobic bacteria PP	Facultative bacteria Gram-negative enterics	Facultative bacteria Streptococci	Facultative bacteria Staphylococci
Cefoxitin-doxycycline	89.76	+++	+++	+++	+++	+++	+++	+++	++
Cefotetan-doxycycline	53.90	+++	+++	+++	+++	+++	+++	+++	++
Ceftizoxime-doxycycline	72.47	+++	+++	+++	+++	+++	+++	+++	++
Cefotaxime-doxycycline	70.97	+++	+++	+++	+++	+++	+++	+++	++
Clindamycin-gentamicin	55.68	++	++	++	+++	+++	+++	++	++
Clindamycin-tobramycin	67.59	++	++	++	+++	+++	+++	++	++
Clindamycin-amikacin	133.19	++	++	++	+++	+++	+++	++	++
Metronidazole-doxycycline	31.49	+	+	+++	+++	+++	+	+	+
Ciprofloxacin	19.12	+++	+++	+	+	+	+++	+	++
Ofloxacin (inpatient)	55.80	+++	+++	+	+	+	+++	+	++
Ofloxacin (outpatient)	5.93								
Sulbactam-ampicillin-doxycycline	54.40	+++	++	+++	++	++	++	++	++
Amoxicillin-clavulanic acid-doxycycline (outpatient)	20.94	+++	++	+++	++	++	++	++	++
Cefoxitin-probenecid-doxycycline (outpatient)	2.64	+++	+++	+++	+++	+++	+++	+++	++

* +++, excellent activity; ++, good activity; +, some activity; PP, penicillinase-producing.
† Price includes pharmacy and administration costs.

antimicrobial regimens for which there were at least three separate trials (Table 5.8). Statistical significance was set at $p \leq 0.005$. Of note, the clinical response rate to penicillin regimens was only 84.1% and to tetracycline alone was 84.5%. On the other hand, the "newer" regimens (i.e., clindamycin plus an aminoglycoside, an extended spectrum cephalosporin plus doxycycline or single-agent therapy with an extended spectrum cephalosporin) had a clinical response rate of 92.9% ($p < 0.001$). Ten of the regimens in Table 5.8 had clinical response rates $\geq$ 90%. Of these regimens, six (clindamycin plus aztreonam, cefoxitin plus doxycycline, ticarcillin plus clavulanic acid, moxalactam, clindamycin plus an aminoglycoside, and cefoxitin alone) had clinical cure rates $\geq$ 90% in at least three published studies and were significantly more effective than tetracycline, penicillin, and penicillin combinations. Dodson[48] reported a significant difference between those antimicrobial regimens with good anaerobic coverage compared with regimens that provide suboptimal anaerobic coverage (93.2% vs. 84.0%; $p < 0.001$). Such data emphasize the importance of including an agent effective against anaerobic bacteria, especially *Prevotella* spp. and

TABLE 5.8. Summary of the efficacy of antimicrobial regimens for the treatment of acute PID.[a]

Drugs	No. of trials	Total no. of patients	No. of patients cured	Clinical response rate (%)
** Clindamycin-aztreonam	3	100	98	98.0
Piperacillin	3	60	57	95.0
** Cefoxitin-doxycycline	6	210	199	94.8
* Imipenem	3	132	125	94.7
** Ticarcillin-clavulanic acid	5	246	232	94.3
** Moxalactam	5	135	127	94.1
* Cefotetan	6	291	271	93.1
** Clindamycin-aminoglycoside	12	374	342	91.4
** Cefoxitin	10	346	315	91.0
Ampicillin-sulbactam	4	92	83	90.2
Metronidazole-aminoglycoside	3	67	59	88.1
† Tetracycline	6	560	473	84.5
‡ Penicillin/ampicillin or Penicillin plus an aminoglycoside, tetracycline or metronidazole	15	726	609	83.9
‡ Older antimicrobial regimens Penicillin and/or ampicillin Pen-aminoglycoside Pen-tetracycline Tetracycline	21	1,286	1,082	84.1
Total Study		4,128	3,711	89.9

* Statistically significantly better than ‡
** Statistically significantly better than † or ‡

[a] Reprinted with permission from Dodson, MG. *J Reprod Med* 1994;**39**:285–296.

Bacteroides fragilis in antimicrobial regimens utilized for the treatment of acute PID.

C. trachomatis is the most common STD organism in the United States.[6] Because of its high prevalence and frequent association with PID, antibiotic coverage of *C. trachomatis*, is included by the CDC in its treatment guidelines for acute PID.[1,6] While in Dodson's review no statistically significant difference was present when comparing single-agent cephalosporin (no coverage for chlamydia) with regimens that cover *C. trachomatis*, such as cefoxitin plus tetracycline or clindamycin plus an aminoglycoside or aztreonam, he proposed several factors that warrant inclusion of an antichlamydial agent in regimens for treatment of acute PID.[48] These include: (1) high prevalence of *C. trachomatis* in patients with acute PID; (2) persistent infection with untreated *C. trachomatis*; and (3) association of chlamydial infection with adverse sequelae such as infertility and/or ectopic pregnancy. Moreover, Sweet et al. noted that *C. trachomatis* persisted in the endometrial cavity of women with PID who had clinically responded to single agent cephalosporins.

In addition to the polymicrobial etiology of PID, clinicians need to recognize that microbial resistance to antibiotics is continuing to increase. National surveillance data has demonstrated increasing resistance of *N. gonorrhoeae* to penicillin, tetracycline, spectinomycin, and cefoxitin.[49] In addition, many of the aerobic and anaerobic bacteria involved in the etiology of PID are increasingly becoming resistant to antibiotics that were commonly used to treat acute PID. Eschenbach[50] reported B-lactamase production by 26% of gram-positive and 17% of gram-negative aerobes recovered from patients with PID. Among anaerobic bacteria, B-lactamases were produced by 37% of gram-positive and 20% of gram-negative organisms (51). In addition, Hasselquist and Hillier[51] demonstrated that the majority of aerobic and anaerobic bacteria recovered from the upper genital tract of PID patients were resistant to tetracycline and doxycycline.

Adequate treatment of acute PID requires evaluation and appropriate treatment of sex partner(s). The CDC recommends that sex partners of women with acute PID should be treated empirically for presumptive infection with *C. trachomatis* and uncomplicated *N. gonorrhoeae*.[6] Table 5.9 provides the recommended regimens for the management of male sex partners of women with acute PID. Treating sexual partners is absolutely essential as demonstrated by a surveillance study of gonococcal PID performed by our group in San Francisco in which 13% of male partners screened were asymptomatic urethral carriers of *N. gonorrhoeae* (Sweet RL, unpublished data). Eschenbach et al.[50] reported that 25% of gonococcal PID patients were admitted to the hospital with a subsequent episode within 10 weeks of initial treatment. Similar and even higher rates of asymptomatic chlamydial urethritis in males also occur. Because the women with acute PID return to the same environment from which they

TABLE 5.9. Management of sex partners of women with acute PID.

Infection	Recommended regimen	Alternative regimens
Chlamydia trachomatis infection	Doxycline 100 mg p.o. b.i.d. × 7 days	Ofloxcine 300 mg p.o. b.i.d. × 7 days
	Azithromycin 1 g p.o. once	Erythromycin base 500 mg or ethylsuccinate 800 mg q.i.d. × 7 days
		Sulfisoxazole 500 mg q.i.d. × 10 days
	PLUS	
Neisseria gonorrhoeae infection	Ceftrixaone 125 mg i.m. once	Spectinomycin 2 g i.m. once
	Cefixime 400 mg p.o. once	Ceftizoxime 500 mg i.m.once
	Ofloxacin 400 mg p.o. once	Cefotaxime 500 mg i.m. once
	Ciprofloxacin 500 mg p.o. once	Cefotetan 1 g i.m. once
		Cefoxitin 1 g i.m. once
		Cefuroxime axetil 1 g p.o. once
		Cefpodoxime proxetil 200 mg p.o. once
		Enoxacin 460 mg p.o. once
		Lomefloxacin 400 mg p.o. once
		Norfloxacin 800 mg p.o. once

came prior to treatment, if the large pool or male partners with asymptomatic STDs are not treated, these women will then be exposed to reinfection and additional episodes of PID.

References

1. Centers for Disease Control. Pelvic inflammatory disease: Guidelines for prevention and management. *MMWR* 1991;**40**:1–25.
2. Wølner-Hanssen P. Silent pelvic inflammatory disease: Is it overstated? *Obstet Gynecol* 1995;**86**:321–325.
3. Viberg L. Acute inflammatory conditions of the uterine adnexa. *Acta Obstet Gynecol Scand* 1964;**43**(S4):5.
4. Swenson CE, Donegan E, Schachter J. *Chlamydia trachomatis* induced salpingitis in mice. *J Infect Dis* 1983;**148**:1101–1107.
5. Swenson CE, Schachter J. Infertility as a consequence of chlamydial infection of the upper genital tract in female mice. *Sex Transm Dis* 1984;**11**:64–67.
6. Centers for Disease Control. 1993 Sexually transmitted disease. Treatment guidelines. *MMWR* 1993;**42**:1–102.
7. Eschenbach DA, Buchanan T, Pollock HM, et al. Polymicrobial etiology of acute pelvic inflammatory disease. *N Engl J Med* 1975;**293**:166.
8. Eschenbach DA, Hillier S, Critchlow C, et al. Diagnosis and clinical manifestations of bacterial vaginosis. *Am J Obstet Gynecol* 1988;**158**:819–828.
9. Rice PA, Schachter J. Pathogenesis of pelvic inflammatory disease caused by *Chlamydia trachomatis* and *Neisseria gonorrhoeae*: Where should research efforts focus? in *Joint Meeting of the Centers for Disease Control and National*

Institutes of Health about Pelvic Inflammatory Disease Prevention, Management, and Research in the 1990's, Bethesda, Maryland, September 4–5, 1990.

10. Paavonen J, Teisala K, Heinonnen PK, et al. Microbiological and his-topathological findings in acute pelvic inflammatory disease. *Br J Obstet Gynecol* 1987;**94**:454–460.

11. Hillier SL, Kiviat NB, Critchlow C, et al. Bacterial vaginosis-associated bacteria as etiologic agents of pelvic inflammatory disease (abstract). *Proceedings of the annual meeting Infectious Disease Society of Obstetrics and Gynecology*. San Diego, CA, August 6, 1992.

12. Sweet RL. Role of bacterial vaginosis in pelvic inflammatory disease. *Clin Infect Dis* 1995;20(suppl 2).

13. Glatt AE, McCormack WM, Taylor Robinson D. Genital mycoplasmas, in Holmes KK, Mardh P-A, Sparling PF, Wiesner PJ (eds): *Sexually Transmitted Diseases*, 2nd ed. New York, McGraw-Hill Information Services, 1990, pp 279–293.

14. Rice PA, Schachter J. Pathogenesis of pelvic inflammatory disease. *JAMA* 1991;**266**:2587–2593.

15. Jossens MOR, Schachter J, Sweet RL. Risk factors associated with pelvic inflammatory disease of differing microbial etiologies. *Obstet Gynecol* 1994;**83**:989–997.

16. Sweet RL. Diagnosis and treatment of acute salpingitis. *J Reprod Med* 1977;**19**:21.

17. Platt R, Rice PA, McCormack WM. Risk of acquiring gonorrhea and preva-lence of abnormal adnexal findings among women recently exposed to gonor-rhea. *JAMA* 1983;**250**:3205–3209.

18. Stamm WE, Guinan ME, Johnson C, et al. Effect of treatment regimens for *Neisseria gonorrhoeae* on simultaneous infection with *Chlamydia trachomatis*. *N Engl J Med* 1984;**310**:545–549.

19. Holtz F. Klinische Studien uber die nicht tuberjulose salpingoophoritis. *Acta Obstet Gynecol* 1930;**10**(S):5.

20. Curtis AH. Bacteriology and pathology of fallopian tubes removed at opera-tion. *Surg Gynecol Obstet* 1921;**33**:621.

21. Andrews FT. Notes on causes of salpingitis. *Am J Obstet Gynecol* 1940; **49**:177.

22. Curtis AH. *Obstetrics and Gynecology*, vol 2. Philadelphia, WB Saunders, 1933, p 497.

23. Falk V. Treatment of acute nontuberculous salpingitis with antibiotics along and in combination with glucocorticoids. *Acta Obstet Gynecol Scand* 1965; **44**(S-16):65.

24. Hedberg E, Anberg A. Gonorrheal salpingitis: Views on treatment and prog-nosis. *Fertil Steril* 1965;**16**:125.

25. Falk V, Krook G. Do results of culture of gonococci vary with sampling phase of menstrual cycle? *Acta Derm Venereol* (Stockh) 1967;**47**:190.

26. Weström LV, Berger GS. Consequences of pelvic inflammatory disease, in Berger GS, Weström LV (eds): Pelvic Inflammatory Disease. New York, Raven Press, 1992, pp 101–114.

27. Hubscher K. Uber die haufgkeit von konzeptionen nach knoservierend und konservativer behandlung von adnexentzundungen. *Zentralbl Gynakol* 1933; **57**:2061–2065.

28. Haffner JC. Resultatene av den konservative og operative salpingitt-behandling. *Nord Med* 1939;**3**:2255–2260.
29. Hedberg E, Spetz SO. Acute salpingitis. Views on prognosis and treatment. *Acta Obstet Gynecol Scand* 1958;**37**:131–135.
30. Weström LV. Incidence, prevalence, and trends of acute pelvic inflammatory disease and its consequences in industrialized countries. *Am J Obstet Gynecol* 1980;**138**:880.
31. Weström LV. Reproductive events after acute salpingitis. *Br J Clin Pract* 1982;**17**(suppl):17–20.
32. Brunham RC, Binns B, Guijon F, et al. Etiology and outcome of acute pelvic inflammatory disease. *J Infect Dis* 1988;**158**:510–517.
33. Safrin S, Schachter J, Dahrouge D, Sweet R. Long-term sequelae of acute pelvic inflammatory disease. *Am J Obstet Gynecol* 1992;**166**:1300–1305.
34. Brunham RC, Binns B, Guijon F, et al. Etiology and outcome of acute pelvic inflammatory disease. *J Infect Dis* 1988;**158**:510–517.
35. Weström LV, Joesoef R, Reynolds G, et al. Pelvic inflammatory disease and fertility. A cohort study of 1,844 women with laparoscopically verified disease and 657 control women with normal laparoscopic results. *Sex Transm Dis* 1992;**19**:185–192.
36. Weström L. Effect of acute pelvic inflammatory disease on fertility. *Am J Obstet Gynecol* 1975;**122**:876.
37. Weström L, Iosif S, Svensson L, et al. Infertility after antibiotics. *Curr Ther* 1979;**26**:752–759.
38. Svensson L, Mardh P-A, Weström L. Infertility after acute salpingitis with special reference to *Chlamydia trachomatis*. *Fertil Steril* 1983;**40**:322–329.
39. Hillis SD, Joesoef R, Marchbanks PA, Wasserheit JN, Willard C, Weström L. Delayed care of pelvic inflammatory disease as a risk factor for impaired fertility. *Am J Obstet Gynecol* 1993;**168**:1503–1509.
40. Katz BP, Zwickl BW, Caine VA, Jones RB. Compliance with antibiotic therapy for *Chlamydia trachomatis* and *Neisseria gonorrhoeae*. *Sex Trans Dis* 1992;**19**:351–354.
41. Sweet RL, Schachter J, Landers DV, et al. Treatment of hospitalized patients with acute pelvic inflammatory disease. Comparison of cefotetan plus doxycycline and cefoxotin plus doxycycline. *Am J Obstet Gynecol* 1988;**158**:736–743.
42. Mourod A, Sweet RL, Sugg N, Schachter J. Relative resistance to erythromycin in *Chlamydia trachomatis*. *Antimicrob Agents Chemother* 1980;**18**:696–698.
43. Wasserheit JN, Bell TA, Kiviat NB, et al. Microbial causes of proven pelvic inflammatory disease and efficacy of clindamycin and tobramycin. *Ann Intern Med* 1986;**104**:187–193.
44. Sweet RL, Schachter J. Ohm-Smith M, et al. Treatment of acute PID: Cefoxitin plus doxycycline versus clindamycin plus tobramycin. Abstract. in *25th Interscience and Conference Antimicrobial Agents Chemotherapy*. Minneapolis, September 29–October 2, 1983.
45. Draper DL, James JF, Hadley WK, Sweet RL. Auxotypes and antibiotic susceptibilities of *Neisseria gonorrhoeae* from women with acute salpingitis. Comparison with gonococci causing uncomplicated genital tract infections in women. *Sex Transm Dis* 1981;**8**:43.
46. Reed SD, Landers DV, Sweet RL. Antibiotic treatment of tubo-ovarian abscess: Comparison of broad spectrum betalactam agents versus clindamycin containing regimens. *Am J Obstet Gynecol* 1991;**164**:1556–1562.

47. Walker CK, Kahn JG, Washington AE, Peterson HB, Sweet RL. Pelvic inflammatory disease. Meta-analysis of antimicrobial regimen efficacy. *J Infect Dis* 1993;**168**:969–978.
48. Dodson MG. Antibiotic regimens for treating acute pelvic inflammatory disease: An evaluation. *J Reprod Med* 1994;**39**:285–296.
49. Schwarcz SK, Zenilman JM, Schnell D, et al. National surveillance of antimicrobial resistance in *Neisseria gonorrhoeae. JAMA* 1990;**264**:1213–1216.
50. Eschenbach DA. A review of beta-lactamase producing bacteria in obstetric-gynecologic infection. *Am J Obstet Gynecol* 1987;**156**:495–498.
51. Hasselquist MB, Hillier S. Susceptibility of upper-genital tract isolates from women with pelvic inflammatory disease to ampicillin, cefpodoxime, metronidazole, and doxycycline. *Sex Transm Dis* 1991;**18**:146–149.

6
Tubo-Ovarian Abscess Complicating Pelvic Inflammatory Disease

Daniel V. Landers

Pelvic Inflammatory Disease (PID) usually involves infection of the endometrial cavity, the fallopian tubes, and the pelvic peritoneal cavity. The proximity of the ovary to the distal fallopian tube places it at risk for infection from adjacent infected structures; particularly at the time of ovulation, which may provide a portal of entry for organisms to gain access to the ovarian stroma. When infection extends beyond the fallopian tube to involve the ovary, the resultant inflammatory response may isolate and wall-off the distal fallopian tube and ovary. As the normal architecture of the fallopian tube and ovary is destroyed in the host's attempt to localize the infection, the result is frequently a sizable tubo-ovarian abscess (TOA). In one series a TOA was identified in 34% of women hospitalized with acute PID although the incidence of TOA has been reported to range from 15% to 34%.[1,2] Because the incidence of TOA is reported as the percent of hospitalized PID patients with TOAs, the reported incidence vary widely depending on how frequently PID patients are hospitalized for treatment.

While no clearly defined risk factors have been identified among women with PID who develop TOA, a good deal of attention has been focused in the past on the intrauterine device (IUD). Some of the earlier retrospective studies in the 1970s reported prior IUD usage in 20% to 54% of women with TOA.[3-5] Several more studies published in the 1980s have found no such association.[1,6,7]

While there seems to be a general assumption that the more episodes of PID the more likely an individual will develop a TOA, studies indicate that over 50% of women with TOA had no prior history of PID.[1,6,8-10] This implies that either a TOA can develop rapidly during the initial episode of PID, or subclinical infection may progress silently to involve the distal fallopian tube and ovary. The latter scenario is similar to women with tubal factor infertility where significant scarring and adhesions are found despite the women having no history of clinically apparent PID.

94

Pathogenesis

Numerous factors play a role in abscess formation including: exotoxins with tissue necrotizing potential; enzymes such as collagenase and heparinase; and virulence factors associated with bacterial capsular polysaccharide.[11] Bacterial antigens also stimulate an inflammatory immune response involving immune cell infiltrates and potentially destructive cytokine synthesis, both of which may contribute to the initial alteration of the upper genital tract morphology. The exact mechanism of TOA formation is difficult to establish, however, both chlamydial and gonococcal salpingitis have been associated with damage to the fallopian tube epithelium. A purulent exudate may develop from this endosalpinx damage. Initially the purulent exudate may spill from the fimbriated end of the fallopian tubes. The ovaries and other pelvic structures may become involved in the inflammatory process during the initial phase of the infection or during a recurrent infection.

There are probably a number of stages in the development of TOA or variations of the same pathogenic mechanism that results in TOA. Pus and adhesion formation may occlude the distal end of the fallopian tube and lead to the development of a pyosalpinx (abscess of the fallopian tube), which spares the ovary. In the earlier stages of TOA development, adjacent pelvic structures such as ometum, bowel, and bladder may adhere to the tube and ovary with filmy or dense adhesion forming a so-called tubo-ovarian complex. It is not clear whether tubo-ovarian complex is an early stage in TOA formation or if it is the endstage of a parallel process involving different patterns or concentrations of microflora reacting to differing host responses.

Microorganisms presumably enter the ovary at an ovulation site, with subsequent tissue invasion. Tissue planes are eventually lost, and the separation of tube and ovary is obscured as the abscess forms. The abscess may remain localized, with involvement of tube and ovary alone, or spread to involve other contiguous pelvic structures, such as bowel, bladder, or the opposite adnexa. An encapsulation process takes place in which the abscess wall serves to localize microbial enzymes or toxins injurious to the host. The development of a dense abscess wall with concurrent destruction of the normal fallopian tube and ovarian architecture represents the final stage in the formation of a TOA. The abscess wall is able to contain those injurious factors and sequester them away from vital structures. The abscess is filled with pus, a neutrophil-rich, inflammatory, viscous, turbid exudate with a pH < 7.0, containing high concentrations of intracellular ions. Immunoglobulins and complement are degraded by the proteolytic enzyme-rich environment of abscess fluid. At any point in the progression, rupture may occur, exposing the peritoneal surface and other intra-abdominal organs to pus, and to myriad pathogens in the case of an untreated abscess. This process can lead to overwhelming sepsis and further abscess formation.

Diagnosis

Standardized diagnostic criteria for TOA do not exist. The clinical diagnosis of TOA suffers the same difficulties and inaccuracies as PID. Women presenting with a clinical diagnosis of PID and a pelvic mass may have a true TOA or may have a pyosalpinx, hydrosalpinx, tubo-ovarian complex, or other simple or complex adnexal masses.

The majority of patients with surgically confirmed TOA will have presented with abdominal and/or pelvic pain, temperature >38.5°C and leukocytosis.[1,12] However, a significant proportion of women with TOA may even have normal temperatures (20% to 30%) and white blood cell counts (WBCs).[1] This may relate to either the stage of disease or conditions in the host. For example, the clinical presentation may be masked if the abscess is completely walled off or in immunosuppressed women less capable of mounting an immune response.

Several laboratory tests may contribute to improved diagnostic accuracy. The erythrocyte sedimentation rate (ESR) has been associated with inflammation and has been used to evaluate severity of infection. Erythrocyte sedimentation rate elevations often lag behind the inflammatory damage and continue to rise as the infection is resolving. The usefulness of ESR as a predictor of the severity of inflammation and long-term sequelae has yet to be documented. More recently, investigators have studied the acute-phase reactant, serum C-reactive protein (CRP) as a diagnostic indicator for tubo-ovarian abscess. It has been found to be more sensitive than elevation in either ESR or white blood cell counts.[13] While this data has yet to be confirmed in large numbers, Mercer and associates[14] showed daily CRP determinations can be used to predict resolution of tubo-ovarian abscess. Further studies are needed to assess the value of CRP as a diagnostic predictor of TOA.

Imaging Techniques

High-resolution imaging techniques have significantly impacted the diagnosis of TOA. The least costly and most frequently used imaging modality is ultrasonography, which provides a reasonably accessible tool to document the presence and complexity of an adnexal mass and to monitor response to therapy. The accuracy of ultrasound in the diagnosis of pelvic abscesses has been evaluated in multiple retrospective studies.[15-20] In one study involving 220 patients with surgically proven abdominal or pelvic abscesses, 36 of 40 abdominal and 32 of 33 pelvic abscesses were correctly identified, while 112 of 113 suspected abdominal and 33 of 34 suspected pelvic abscesses were correctly ruled out.[16]

In another series, 98 TOA patients were studied with ultrasound of which 31 had surgically confirmed TOA. They found 29 of 31 surgically confirmed tubo-ovarian abscesses were correctly diagnosed using ultrasound. The presence of a mass was identified in 100% of surgically confirmed TOAs and in 90% of the 67 clinically diagnosed TOA patients.[1] The expected typical appearance of a tubo-ovarian abscess on ultrasound is a complex or cystic adnexal mass with multiple internal echoes (Figure 6.1). While unilocular abscesses can appear as thick-walled cysts, most often some internal echoes and/or loculations can be identified.

Ultrasound has also been used to follow resolution of abscesses managed conservatively. As the field of ultrasound continues to be refined, the usefulness of this tool will be even greater in this regard. Presently, ultrasound is the least expensive approach to imaging the pelvis and has a diagnostic sensitivity of at least 90% in identifying pelvic abscesses.

Computed tomography (CT) scans have been used extensively in the diagnosis and treatment of intra-abdominal abscesses (Figure 6.2). Data on the accuracy of CT scans in the diagnosis of tubo-ovarian abscess is scant. One study evaluating the accuracy of ultrasound, gallium scans, and CT scans in the diagnosis of abdominal abscesses reported the sensitivity of ultrasound, gallium, and CT as 82%, 96%, and 100%, respectively.[21] Specificity was reported as 91%, 65%, and 100%, respectively for these techniques. In a more recent study, Jasinsky[19] compared the sensitivity of ultrasound with CT scan in the diagnosis of intra-abdominal, including pelvic abscesses. In this study, the sensitivity of ultrasound was 42/56 (75%) and CT scan was 14/15 (93%) for pelvic abscesses, the differences being

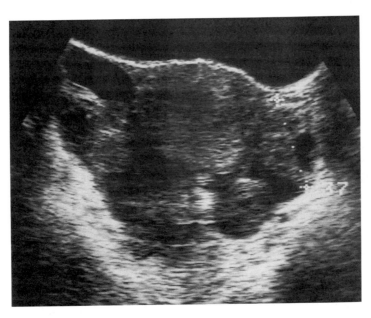

Figure 6.1. Transverse sonographic image of centrally located uterus and bilateral tubo-ovarian abscesses.

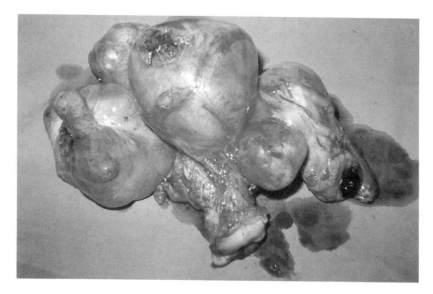

FIGURE 6.2. Surgical specimen of bilateral tubo-ovarian abscesses immediately following extirpation.

attributed to difficulties in ultrasound evaluation of postoperative oncology patients. Thus, CT scans appear to be accurate in detecting the presence of intra-abdominal abscesses. There is less data available concerning CT evaluation of pelvic abscesses but it does seem quite accurate. In view of the expense, CT scans should generally be reserved for situations where ultrasound studies with vaginal probe fail to provide sufficient information.

Magnetic resonance imaging (MRI) has certainly proven to be a valuable tool for diagnostic imaging. It has the advantages of being capable of discriminating between differing contiguous tissue densities and doing so without the use of ionizing radiation. Unfortunately, it remains quite expensive and lacks sufficient data demonstrating superior diagnostic capabilities in the diagnosis of TOA. It remains to be seen whether clinical experience with MRI will confirm the theoretical advantages in differentiating pelvic masses, particularly in the setting of an abscess. It will further be necessary to show significant advantages over ultrasound to justify the added expense.

Microbiology

The microbiology reported in the majority of TOA studies may be somewhat misleading. Frequently, cultures of the abscess are obtained long after antibiotic agents have been administered. This may well suppress the growth if not prevent isolation of any number of potential pathogens. Furthermore, the resistant gram-negative anaerobic organisms with polysaccharide capsules capable of inducing the type of immune response that leads to abscess formation may not be identified unless strict anaerobic isolation, transport, and culture techniques are used. Studies utilizing these techniques have shown that anaerobic organisms are the most prevalent isolates from TOAs, having been recovered from 63% to 100% of adnexal abscesses.[1,22–26] The concept of a sterile abscess may well represent an abscess in which poor anaerobic collection and culture techniques prevented the isolation of organisms or where the antimicrobial agents have gained access to the abscess cavity prior to obtaining the culture. In our studies at San Francisco General Hospital in the 1970s and early 1980s, the predominant organisms isolated from TOAs were *Escherichia coli*, *Bacteroides fragilis*, other *Bacteroides* species, aerobic streptococci, and *peptostreptococcus* species.[1] While it is uncommon to isolate *Neisseria gonorrhoeae* or *Chlamydia trachomatis* from a TOA, these organisms, in particular *N. gonorrhoeae*, have been implicated in the initial penetration of the endocervical barrier leading to anaerobic invasion of the upper genital tract. The facultative and anaerobic organisms may later suppress the growth of *N. gonorrhoeae*, preventing recovery. Animal studies have shown that, while encapsulated *Bacteroides* species will lead to subcutaneous abscess formation, this effect can be synergistically enhanced with *N. gonorrhoeae*, particularly when encapsulated. Even when *N. gonorrhoeae* and *Bacteroides* species were used in combination and abscess formation occurred, recovery of *N. gonorrhoeae* from the abscess was not possible after the seventh day.[27] The counts of *Bacteroides* isolates, however, were greater in the abscesses if also inoculated with *N. gonorrhoeae*.

It has become increasingly clear that a significant portion of women with PID are not infected with either *C. trachomatis* or *N. gonorrhoeae*. In these women, potential pathogens found in the lower genital tract, particularly the anaerobes, may invade the upper genital tract. The emergence and recognition of *Prevotella bivia* (formerly *Bacteroides bivius*) and *Prevotella disiens* as major pathogens in upper female genital tract infection combined with data suggesting that increased concentration of anaerobic organisms in the vagina is a risk factor for PID both point toward an anaerobe predominant mixed infection as a cause of PID. This type of PID may represent a group of women more susceptible to TOA formation.

A less common organism that has been reported in association with TOA is *Actinomyces israelii*, a gram-positive aerobe. In one report, 7/8 (88%) of PID patients with actinomycetes has TOAs compared with 11/38 (29%) without TOA.[28] This organism also has been reported in association with IUD use.[29,30] The exact role of this organism in the pathogenesis of TOA is unclear because it has not been recovered in the vast majority of TOA patients studied over the years.

Treatment

The vast majority of intra-abdominal abscesses are effectively treated with a combination of antimicrobial therapy and drainage. Success with medical therapy alone has been reported in several types of abscesses including brain, liver, and TOAs. These sites all share the common feature of a rich vascular supply by which effective antimicrobial agents can be efficiently delivered to the abscess site.

Whether or not combining medical therapy with drainage in the treatment of TOAs improves the outcome remains controversial. Reports of success using this combined approach have been nonrandomized studies without a control group receiving antimicrobials alone.[31-33] These studies report a remarkably high cure rate and shortened hospital courses over historical controls. One should exercise some caution in interpreting these studies. Selection bias in determining candidates for drainage and/or inclusion of patients with "tubo-ovarian complexes" may lead to spurious conclusions. Furthermore, there is no information available concerning future fertility in women undergoing drainage procedures compared with those treated with antimicrobial agents alone.

In this section we will discuss the various treatment modalities including antimicrobial agents, approaches to drainage, and surgical extirpation of TOAs with and without hysterectomy.

Antimicrobial Agents

Selection of antimicrobial agents in the treatment of TOA should be based on the nature of this process. Broad spectrum agents or combinations of agents should be used with particular attention to anaerobic coverage. The overall initial success rate in treating TOA with well-selected antimicrobial agents has been reported to be as high as 86%.[1] The mean rate of success in recent studies has been in the range of 70% to 75% when regimens including coverage for the resistant gram-negative anaerobic bacteria were used.[2,34,35-37] The success rates in using antimicrobial agents alone will vary significantly depending on a number of factors. The size of the abscess and whether or not there are bilateral abscesses have both been associated with the need for surgical intervention.[1,34] An increasing temperature and/or WBC in the face of antimicrobial therapy also have been predictive of medical treatment failure.[1]

The choice of antimicrobials for the treatment of TOA should be based on the likely organisms present rather than what might be cultured from pus or the abscess wall. Many of the organisms responsible for this condition are difficult to isolate without specialized anaerobic culture and transport techniques. The most studied antimicrobials for the treatment of abscesses have been clindamycin and metronidazole. These agents have been studied extensively in *in vitro* systems, animal models, and human clinical trials. The gold standard for the treatment of TOA has been a combination of clindamycin and an aminoglycoside such as gentamicin. Many other combinations of antimicrobial agents have been studied in the treatment of TOA but none shown to be superior to the clindamycin/gentamicin combination, which is also one of the Centers for Disease Control (CDC) recommended combinations for the inpatient treatment of PID. Our preference for treatment of known TOA is a combination that includes clindamycin or metronidazole based on their superior ability to penetrate and remain active inside the abscess. Frequently the presence of a TOA is discovered after antimicrobial therapy has begun for PID. Because the combination of cefoxitin or cefotetan with doxycycline is commonly used to treat inpatient PID, the question that often arises is whether these patients should be switched to a clindamycin-containing regimen or should clindamycin be added to the regimen. We have found that although there may be a theoretical advantage to this approach, it does not seem to change the outcome in terms of the need for surgical intervention.[34] Thus, if patients are discovered to have a TOA while on a CDC recommended inpatient PID regimen and are responding clinically, we generally will continue this course of therapy unless the need for surgical intervention arises. We do recommend that all patients with TOA be treated for a full 7 days of parenteral antimicrobials to optimize the chance of resolving the abscess without the need for surgical intervention. We continue to await results of randomized trials comparing antimicrobials alone with antimicrobials plus early laparoscopic drainage in terms of cure rates, length of hospital stay, and long-term outcome with regard to the need for further surgery and fertility prognosis.

Surgical Intervention

Indications for surgical intervention in the treatment of PID complicated by TOA include: (1) questionable diagnoses where another surgical emergency may exist (e.g., appendicitis); (2) rupture of the abscess; and (3) failure of medical therapy with or without a drainage procedure.

The first two indications generally constitute the need for immediate surgical intervention. Questionable diagnoses in which another surgical emergency is a serious consideration is commonly approached by diagnostic laparoscopy or exploratory laparotomy. Intraperitoneal rupture of a TOA represents a true surgical emergency. Delayed intervention may increase the risk of septic shock and even death. There is general agreement that acute rupture of a TOA requires immediate surgery, however the extent of surgery necessary to affect a cure remains controversial. Aggressive antimicrobial therapy combined with unilateral adnexectomy has been shown to be safe and effective management for a ruptured unilateral TOA in women who want to maintain their reproductive and hormonal capacities.

The unruptured TOA may also require surgical intervention when anti-microbial agents fail to illicit a favorable acute response or the abscess persists after the acute inflammatory phase. A number of surgical proce-dures have been used as primary or adjunctive therapy in treatment of unruptured TOAs. The posterior colpotomy was used for years to effect drainage of abscesses accessible through the posterior vagina. This proce-dure is most effective when the abscess dissects to the lower one-third of the rectovaginal septum. The posterior colpotomy has been largely abandoned because of the high rate of complications and frequent need for additional surgery. When performed, it is essential that the abscess be adherent to the pelvic parietal peritoneum to prevent intra-abdominal leakage. Colpotomy drainage of TOAs has largely been replaced by either drainage under direct visualization through the laparoscope or laparotomy with extirpation of the entire abscess.

Because as many as 70% of TOAs are reportedly unilateral, the majority of those not responding to antimicrobials alone can be surgically managed without removing the uterus or opposite adnexa. Even in the case of bilat-eral disease there may be reason to avoid hysterectomy, particularly in cases where some ovarian tissue can be preserved. The advantages of conservative surgery include maintaining potential fertility and hormonal function and reducing blood loss, potential for bowel and bladder complica-tions, postoperative complications, and length of hospitalization. There may be other significant advantages as well, such as avoiding the psycho-logical, sexual, and sensory difficulties that some women experience follow-ing hysterectomy.

Technical Considerations

When exploratory surgery is undertaken in women with suspected TOA careful consideration should be given to the size, location, laterality, and complexity of the abscess. Tissue planes may be distorted particularly in the case of ruptured abscess. The dissection may be difficult, bloody and re-quire extensive blunt and sharp dissection to separate contiguous structures such as bowel and bladder from the abscess wall. In choosing the appropri-ate incision, care should be taken to provide adequate exposure. The cosmetically appealing Pfannenstiel incision may not provide adequate exposure for large and/or bilateral TOAs. This incision may predispose to subfascial abscess formation and limit access to the upper abdomen. Low vertical incisions facilitate enlarging the incision, if necessary. The Maylard incision is an option that combines increased exposure with more desirable cosmetics and strength of closure.

Upon entering the abdomen, the entire cavity should be explored, includ-ing the area under the diaphragm, for the presence of free or loculated pockets of purulent material. All collections of purulent material should be gently dispersed, disrupted, or drained. The difficulty of abscess surgery relates to the extent the tissue planes are disrupted, the degree of adhesion formation and the amount of distortion to the normal anatomy. Careful dissection of the abscess from surrounding structures is important to avoid injury to contiguous organs. The ureters must be located and traced from the pelvic brim to their insertions into the bladder prior to extirpation of pelvic structures.

If rupture or leakage of the abscess has occurred, the placement of drains attached to low pressure suction may allow for continued decompression and prevent abscess reformation. When hysterectomy has been performed, the cuff should be left open and a large-bore Malecot drain placed exiting through the vaginal cuff once hemostasis has been achieved. In instances of conservative surgical management, a posterior colopotomy may be used to accommodate one or several Jackson–Pratt drains. In the event that the cul-de-sac is not accessible, drains may be brought out through the abdominal wall through a stab wound separate from the incision. These drains should be removed approximately 48h following surgery.

Before closure, generous irrigation with warm saline is essential to reduce the innoculum or organisms and inflammatory materials. The use of intraperitoneal antibiotics has not proven helpful. Optimal closure of the abdomen can be achieved with a Smead–Jones technique using a synthetic nonabsorbable or long-lasting monofilament suture. If one chooses to irrigate the subcutaneous tissues, warm saline should be utilized instead of antibiotic or providone-iodine solutions, as they have not been shown to reduce the incidence of wound infections. The subcutaneous layer should be closed in a delayed primary fashion. The defect is packed with a moistened find mesh gauze, which is left sterile for a period of approximately 4 days. At that time, the gauze is removed, the incision base inspected, and the skin edges apposed using tapes or sutures if no signs of infection are present.

Fertility Following TOA

Tubo-ovarian abscess management aimed at preserving reproductive organs helps maintain hormonal function but does not assure future fertility. Damage from inflammation and scarring to the fine structure of the fallopian tube as well as gross obstruction significantly impair fertility. Several investigators have reported that approximately 10% (9.5% to 13.8%) of women have subsequent pregnancy following TOAs but follow-up did not include determining how many patients were attempting pregnancy.[1,6,10,38,39] These figures were from women treated with antibiotics alone. The pregnancy rate ranged from 3.7% to 16% following unilateral adnexal procedures with preoperative antibiotics,[1,6,38] and 10% to 15% following antibiotics plus colpotomy drainage.[40–42] Hager recently published a series in which 50 patients treated for TOAs were evaluated.[43] A total of 11 of these patients had reproductive potential following treatment, but only 8 attempted to conceive. Four of the eight (50%) conceived a total of five intrauterine pregnancies. There were no ectopic pregnancies. Included in this group were five patients who underwent unilateral salpingo-oophorectomy and attempted to conceive, of whom four were successful (80%). Thus, we may be underestimating dramatically reproductive potential following TOAs, unless we consider the number of patients attempting to conceive following conservative medical or surgical management. Furthermore, newer antibiotics that are better able to penetrate abscesses may enhance fertility outcome.

Summary

Significant improvement in the management of TOAs has been made over the last 20 to 30 years. The development of broader spectrum antimicrobials with the capacity to penetrate an abscess has provided a viable alternative to surgical extirpation in most cases. Conservative approaches to surgical intervention (when required) have shown also to be successful and beneficial to mental and physiological health of women following TOA. The usefulness of laparoscopic drainage to further enhance outcome needs to be studied prospectively in randomized, controlled studies that include medical management and medical management plus laparoscopic drainage with clinical response, fertility, and ectopic pregnancy as outcome variables.

References

1. Landers DV, Sweet RL. Tubo-ovarian abscess: Contemporary approach to management. *Rev Infect Dis* 1983;**5**:876.
2. Landers DV, Sweet RL. Current trends in the diagnosis and treatment of tuboovarian abscess. *Am J Obstet Gynecol* 1985;**151**:1098.
3. Dawood MY, Birnbaum SJ. Unilateral tuboovarian abscess and an intrauterine contraceptive device. *Obstet Gynecol* 1975;**46**:429.
4. Golditch IM, Huston JE. Serious pelvic infections associated with intrauterine contraceptive devices. *Int J Fertil* 1973;**18**:156.
5. Taylor ES, McMillan JH, Green BE, et al. The intrauterine device. *Obstet Gynecol* 1975;**46**:429.
6. Ginsberg DS, Stern JL, Hamod KA, et al. Tuboovarian abscess: A retrospective review. *Am J Obstet Gynecol* 1980;**138**:1055.
7. Manara LR. Management of tubo-ovarian abscess. *J Am Osteopath Assoc* 1982;**81**:476.
8. Benigno BB. Medical and surgical management of the pelvic abscess. *Clin Obstet Gynecol* 1981;**24**:1187.
9. Edelman DA, Berger GS. Contraceptive practice and tuboovarian abscess. *Am J Obstet Gynecol* 1980;**138**:541.
10. Franklin EW, Hevron JE, Thompson JD. Management of the pelvic abscess. *Clin Obstet Gynecol* 1973;**16**:66.

11. Zaleznik DF, Kasper DL. The role of anaerobic bacteria in abscess formation. *Ann Rev Med* 1982;**38**:217.
12. Mickal A, Sellmann AH. Management of tubo-ovarian abscess. *Clin Obstet Gynecol* 1969;**12**:252.
13. Lehtenen M, Laine S, Heinonnen PK, et al. Serum C-reactive protein determination in acute pelvic inflammatory disease. *Am J Obstet Gynecol* 1986;**154**:158.
14. Mercer LJ, Hajj SM, Ismail MA, et al. Use of creative protein to predict the outcome of medical management of tuboovarian abscesses. *J Reprod Med* 1988;**33**:164.
15. Filly RA. Detection of abdominal abscesses: A combined approach employing ultrasonography, computed tomography and gallium-67 scanning. *J Assoc Can Radiol* 1979;**30**:202.
16. Taylor KJW, DeGraaft MCI, Wasson JF, Rosenfeld AT, Andriole VT. Accuracy of grey-scale ultrasound diagnosis of abdominal and pelvic abscesses in 220 patients. *Lancet* 1978;**1**:83.
17. Spirtos NJ, Bernstine EL, Crawford WL, Fayle J. Sonography in acute pelvic inflammatory disease. *J Reprod Med* 1982;**27**:312.
18. Uhrich PC, Sanders RC. Ultrasonic characteristics of pelvic inflammatory masses. *J Clin Ultrasound* 1976;**4**:199.
19. Jasinsky RW, Glazer GM, Francis IR, et al. CT and ultrasound in abscess detection at specific anatomic sites: A study of 198 patients. *Comput Radiol* 1987;**11**:41.
20. Ferruci JT Jr, van Sonnonberg E. Intraabdominal abscess: Radiological diagnosis and treatment. *JAMA* 1981;**246**:2728–2733.
21. Moir C, Robins RE. Role of ultrasound, gallium scanning and computed tomography in the diagnosis of intraabdominal abscess. *Am J Surg* 1982;**143**:582.
22. Swenson RM, Michaelson TC, Daly MJ, et al. Anaerobic bacterial infections of the female genital tract. *Obstet Gynecol* 1973;**42**:538.
23. Thadepalli H, Gorbach SL, Keith L. Anaerobic infections of the female genital tract: Bacteriologic and therapeutic aspects. *Am J Obstet Gynecol* 1973;**117**:1034.
24. Altemeier WA. The anaerobic streptococci in tubo-ovarian abscess. *Am J Obstet Gynecol* 1940;**39**:1038.
25. Ledger WJ, Campbell C, Wilson JR. Postoperative adnexal infections. *Obstet Gynecol* 1968;**31**:83.
26. Pearson HE, Anderson GV. Genital bacteroidal abscesses in women. *Am J Obstet Gynecol* 1970;**107**:1264.
27. Brooks I. Metronidazole and spiramycin in abscess caused by *Bacteroides* sp. and *Staphylococcus aureus* in mice. *J Antimicrobial Chemother* 1987;**20**:713.
28. Burkman R, Schelesselman S, McCaffrey L, et al. The relationship of genital tract actinomycetes and the development of pelvic inflammatory diseases. *Am J Obstet Gynecol* 1982;**143**:585.
29. Schiffer MA, Elguezabal A, Sultana M, Allen AC. Actinomycosis infections associated with intrauterine contraceptive devices. *Obstet Gynecol* 1975;**45**:67.
30. Lomax CW, Harbert GM, Thornton WN. Actinomycosis of the female genital tract. *Obstet Gynecol* 1976;**48**:341.
31. Henry-Suchet J, Soler A, Loffredo V. Laparoscopic treatment of tuboovarian abscesses. *J Reprod Med* 1984;**29**:579.

32. Reich H, McGlynn F. Laparoscpic treatment of tuboovarian and pelvic abscess. *J Reprod Med* 1987;**32**:747.
33. Dellenbach P, Mueller P, Philippe E. Infections utero annexielles aigues. *Encycl Med Chir Gynecol* 1972;**470**:1410.
34. Reed SD, Landers DV, Sweet RL. Antibiotic treatment of tuboovarian abscess. *Am J Obstet Gynecol* 1991;**164(6)**:1556.
35. Walters MD, Gibbs RS. A randomized comparison of gentamicin-clindamycin and cefoxitin-doxycycline in the treatment of acute pelvic inflammatory disease. *Obstet Gynecol* 1990;**75**:867.
36. Martens MG, Faro S, Hammill H, et al. Comparison of cefotaxime, cefoxitin, and clindamycin plus gentamicin in the treatment of uncomplicated and complicated pelvic inflammatory disease. *J Antimicrob Chemother* 1990;**26**(suppl A):37.
37. Sweet RL, Schachter J, Landers DV, et al. Treatment of hospitalized patients with acute pelvic inflammatory disease: Comparison of cefotetan plus doxycycline and cefoxitin plus doxycycline. *Am J Obstet Gynecol* 1988;**158**:736.
38. Golde SH, Israel R, Ledger WJ. Unilateral tuboovarian abscess: A distinct entity. *Am J Obstet Gynecol* 1977;**127**:807.
39. Hemsell DC, Santos-Ramos R, Cunningham FG, et al. Cefotaxime treatment for women with community-acquired pelvic abscesses. *Am J Obstet Gynecol* 1985;**151**:171.
40. Rivlin ME. Clinical outcome following vaginal drainage of pelvic abscess. *Obstet Gynecol* 1983;**61**:169.
41. Rivlin ME. Golan A, Darling MR. Diffuse peritoneal sepsis associated with colpotomy drainage of pelvic abscess. *J Reprod Med* 1982;**27**:406.
42. Rivlin ME, Hunt JA. Ruptured tuboovarian abscess: Is hysterectomy necessary? *Obstet Gynecol* 1977;**50**:518.
43. Hager WD. Follow-up of patients with TOA in association with salpingitis. *Obstet Gynecol* 1983;**61**:680.

7
Pelvic Inflammatory Disease in Pregnancy

Joseph G. Pastorek II

> *Things are seldom what they seem,*
> *Skim milk masquerades as cream.*
> H.M.S. Pinafore (Act I)

It is a truism in medicine that the diagnosis that is not sought is the diagnosis that will not be found. Every medical student is taught by his mentors the philosophy of the differential diagnosis, that is, naming every pathological entity that *could* be the cause of a particular patient's disease, and then weeding out, by history, examination, or laboratory study, those which are not. The importance of this initial list of diagnoses, then, is beyond measure; if an illness is not mentioned therein, it will be overlooked. And because many maladies are symptomatically similar to other, unrelated diseases, the physician is compelled to apply much of his intellect to the study of differential diagnosis.

The patient presenting with fever, abdominal pain, and a positive pregnancy test has long been the source of consternation and anxiety to the obstetrician. Especially in the first trimester, this type of patient represents to the physician a true diagnostic dilemma. On the one hand, there appears to be some sort of intra-abdominal catastrophe, perhaps of an infectious nature such as appendicitis. On the other hand, the patient is pregnant and thoughts of ectopic gestation come immediately to mind. To make things more complex, any diagnostic or therapeutic measures must be undertaken cautiously, so as not to harm a possible viable fetus. It is against this backdrop that the question of pelvic inflammatory disease (PID) complicating pregnancy arises. This chapter is an attempt to refute any misperceptions and persuade the reader of the truth of this issue once and for all.

Coexistence of PID and Pregnancy

It should be mentioned at the outset that there is a large cadre of obstetricians and gynecologists, clinical and academic types, who deny that PID and pregnancy can coexist. This results in the immortalization of this

TABLE 7.1. Reported cases of PID and pelvic abscess in pregnancy.

Reference (first author)	PID cases	Abscess cases	Maternal deaths	Fetal deaths
Lennon[3] (1949)	2	0	0	1
McCord[4] (1953)	2	0	0	2
Scott[5] (1954)	2	0	0	2
Lancet[6] (1959)	1	0	0	1
Friedman[2] (1959)	3	2	0	2
Acosta[7] (1971)	4	0	0	2
Jafari[8]* (1977)	0	17	3	8
Fuselier[9] (1978)	0	1	0	0
Stubbs[10] (1985)	0	1	0	1
Davey[11] (1987)	0	1	0	1
Blanchard[12] (1987)	3	0	0	1
Andersen[13] (1988)	1	0	0	?
Kouyoumdjian[14] (1990)	1	0	0	1
Total	19	22	3	22

*Review article that includes reference 2 (numbers of patients appropriately adjusted).

disinformation. In many places, through formal conferences, patient rounds, etc., students and house officers are taught that pregnant women cannot have PID. Articles in standard publications by renowned authors have said, for instance, that the cervical mucous plug, the fetal membranes, and the decidua are barriers to any ascending infection during pregnancy. As well, pelvic hyperemia due to pregnancy tended to prevent or ameliorate such infections.[1] Others have basically dismissed PID in pregnancy as being an "ill-defined subject" and "probably due to criminal interference."[2]

In spite of the widespread bias against the existence of PID in pregnancy, there have steadily, over the years, accumulated case reports and small series of salpingitis and even pelvic abscess complicating pregnancy. Fairly superficial review of the English literature since about 1950 reveals over 40 documented cases of PID and pelvic abscess discovered during pregnancy, not to mention other cases and reports alluded to but poorly documented (Table 7.1). Before 1949, according to one author,[3] cases had only been reported by French gynecologists, who were impressed with their invariable misdiagnosis as appendicitis or ectopic pregnancy. The prevailing thought, at least among English-speaking writers, was that PID did not occur during pregnancy. Rather, patients with the clinical presentation described above either represented spontaneous septic abortion/amnionitis, or were actually suffering the after effects of self-induced, illegal abortion.

What is written in the journals, however, may not always represent the general consensus. In point of fact, one author bluntly states that although the French practitioners wrote of the disease and the English did not, "... PID in pregnancy is an accepted occurrence to most physicians. Despite strong theoretical objections against it and little concrete evidence in favor of it . . ."[2] It would appear that in the earlier literature, there was a strong academic bias against the coexistence of PID and pregnancy on scientific grounds, although the clinical diagnosis was made "casually."[2]

Pathophysiology

Earlier skepticism concerning PID in pregnancy was based upon an assumption, as noted above, that the intact conceptus acted as a barrier to ascending infection. Some authors agreed that PID could occur in early pregnancy, before the layers of the decidua fused to obliterate the endometrial cavity, because that was in keeping with the generally accepted idea that PID was an infection that ascended the genital tract through the endometrial cavity during menses. As early as 1939 though, one French writer advanced a number of other mechanisms whereby microorganisms could reach the upper genital tract during pregnancy.[15] To his list were added other feasible mechanisms[7,12] such that no modern obstetrician should be without ammunition to explain a case of PID (or pelvic abscess) occurring during gestation (Table 7.2, Figure 7.1).

Scientifically speaking, one can ponder the various mechanisms proposed and come to some understanding of the pathophysiology of this condition. It certainly seems reasonable to consider the "usual" mechanism of transuterine spread of pathogenic organisms, for example, the gonococcus, to occur primarily in early gestation before the obliteration of the endometrial cavity. Indeed, many of the undocumented cases referred to in the literature were said to be early and culture-positive for *Neisseria gonorrhoeae*. However, few of the cases documented in Table 7.1 were culture-positive and most were in the middle trimester, contradicting the usual understanding of the condition. It would seem, then, that "early GC PID of pregnancy" is not the usually encountered form of the disease.

TABLE 7.2. Mechanisms of development of PID and pelvic abscess during pregnancy.

Infection occurring at the time of fertilization
Infection occurring soon after fertilization before the uterine cavity has become closed
   (about 12 wks)
Vascular or lymphatic spread
Flare-up of preexisting infection
Instrumentation sufficient to overcome natural barriers
Ascending infection associated with threatened abortion and intrauterine bleeding
Hematogenous dissemination from distant sources
Contiguous spread from adjacent organs

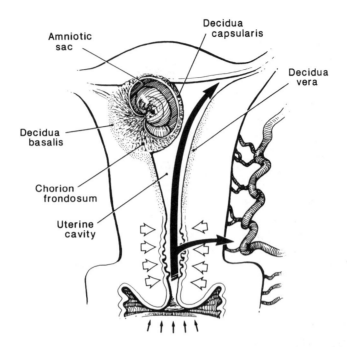

FIGURE 7.1. Mechanisms of bacterial spread from the cervix into the upper genital tract. Small arrows = exposure to bacteria; open arrows = colonized sites in the lower uterus and cervix; solid arrows = transuterine spread and hematogenous and lymphatic spread.

Pelvic abscess, on the other hand, is usually encountered in the middle to later stages of pregnancy. The one large review[8] reported only 3 of 17 patients as being less than 12 wks gestation. Conceptually, it would be easy to imagine that abscesses occur as the result of smoldering infection that has been present for some time, or infection spread from adjacent or distant sources. That is, it is not necessary to posit a transuterine insult to explain the lesion. It should be specifically noted that it is not unusual for abscesses to be discovered at or near term.[8,9,11]

Diagnosis

As the French gynecologists discovered, PID in pregnancy is usually mistaken for other illnesses. Appendicitis and ectopic pregnancy are the two major misdiagnosis encountered in the usual course of practice. Many of the cases in Table 7.1 were in fact diagnosed at laparotomy by physicians expecting to find one of these two entities. For example, the first case from the author's institution[12] underwent surgical exploration for presumed appendicitis, in spite of a positive cervical smear for gram-negative, intracellular diplococci, because of the bias against the possibility of the existence of PID in pregnancy. The reader is left to wonder how many other cases are dismissed because of similar prejudice.

It is imperative that the differential diagnosis of a patient presenting with fever and pain during pregnancy be broad enough to enable the obstetrician to include the correct diagnosis in his evaluation (Table 7.3). Also to this end, it is important to collect the appropriate diagnostic information. The physical examination and history are of paramount importance. Care must be taken to obtain an exact menstrual and sexual history, because pregnancy and sexually transmitted disease are obviously foremost in mind. Complete blood count and differential, urinalysis, gram stain of cervical discharge, and perhaps general chemistry panel (especially for liver functions) are all in order, keeping an eye primarily upon evidence of infection and its location. Ultrasonography, while commonly performed, may actually be worthless if a reasonable pelvic examination has been possible. However, if there is any doubt as to the existence of an intrauterine (vs. extrauterine) pregnancy, in gestations discovered early enough that simple bimanual examination may not detect uterine enlargement, then a sonographic survey of the pelvis may rule in (or rule out) an intrauterine gestational sac.

The physician must at all times keep the possible diagnoses firmly in mind, as the information is accumulated. Neither must any possibility be discarded before it is thoroughly investigated. Too many cases of ectopic pregnancy, for example, have been overlooked because the patient's temperature was "too high," in spite of the fact that free blood in the peritoneal cavity may incite fever. As well, the patient with fever that is "too low" may still harbor an early appendicitis, its symptoms modified by the anti-inflammatory effects of progesterone. In all cases, the practitioner must utilize his keenest judgment, remembering that there is no "classic" case of PID or pelvic abscess in pregnancy.

TABLE 7.3. Differential diagnosis of pain, fever, and pregnancy.

Appendicitis
Bowel obstruction/infarction
Degeneration of leiomyoma
Ectopic pregnancy
Medical illness (e.g., sickle crisis)
Pancreatitis/hepatitis
Pelvic abscess
Pelvic inflammatory disease
Placental abruption
Renal stone/infection
Threatened/incomplete abortion
Torsion of adnexal cyst/tumor

Because the diagnosis in these patients is often problematic, diagnostic laparoscopy is often the ultimate diagnostic method of choice. In recent decades, advances in laparoscopic technique have enabled gynecologists to avoid laparotomy in many cases that would have previously come to more invasive ends. The possibility of surgically correcting a tubal ectopic gestation, as well as the beneficial effects of initiating proper antibiotic therapy for patients with salpingitis, is quite conducive to the use of diagnostic laparoscopy in perplexing cases. The surgeon must beware, however, of overlooking some primary site of infection (e.g., appendicitis) after the pelvis is noted to be uniformly inflamed. The laparoscopy, as a diagnostic procedure, must be performed in its entirety, including visualization of the appendix and other intra-abdominal structures such as the gall bladder.

More complex and novel approaches to diagnosis in cases of pain and fever during pregnancy are not commonly utilized. Computerized tomography of the abdominal structures is not recommended in the presence of a viable fetus. Magnetic resonance imaging, while safe during pregnancy, has not been widely practiced in these circumstances and is likely to be too expensive and unlikely to be of any great benefit over the other diagnostic modalities mentioned (i.e., physical examination and laparoscopy).

Finally, the physician should never succumb to professional arrogance after the tentative diagnosis is made. Pelvic inflammatory disease in pregnancy and all of its mimics are difficult diagnostic dilemmas; misdiagnosis is almost the rule and not the exception. The patient, after appropriate therapy is instituted, should be diligently followed for the possibility that she actually has some other disease entity. This is exceedingly important in cases where the patient's clinical course is not progressing according to plan, that is, the clinical picture over the first couple of days of therapy is not improving as rapidly as expected.

Therapy

Assuming that the diagnosis of PID has been appropriately made, the antibiotic therapy thereof is essentially identical to treatment of PID in the nonpregnant woman and is reviewed elsewhere in this volume. The physician must keep two concepts clearly in mind, though, when treating the pregnant woman with presumed PID:1) The abortion rate is high in such cases,[2-7] leading to the recommendation of rapid initiation of therapy [12] (perhaps even before the physician and any consultants agree upon a diagnosis); and 2) certain antibiotics are relatively contraindicated in pregnant women, due to theoretical or potential adverse effects on the fetus.

Antibiotic therapy of PID generally consists of antibiotic coverage of five groups of organisms: N. gonorrhoeae, Chlamydia trachomatis, anaerobic bacteria (e.g., *Bacteroides* species), gram-negative facultative bacteria (e.g., *Escherichia coli*), and the streptococci.[16] Such coverage may be achieved with a number of therapeutic agents, including β-lactam drugs (i.e., penicillins, cephalosporins), clindamycin/aminoglycoside combinations, tetracyclines (especially extended spectrum tetracyclines such as doxycycline and minocycline), the new quinolone antibiotics (e.g., ofloxicin), and various others.[17] Physicians often follow the Centers for Disease Control guidelines and use a cephalosporin plus doxycycline or the "gold standard" clindamycin/gentamicin combination. However, use of some of these drugs during pregnancy is relatively contraindicated.

Tetracyclines may cause fetal skeletal abnormalities and dental (enamel) hypoplasia if used during gestation, though short courses seem to have little effect.[18] Aminoglycosides, while associated with fetal auditory damage in cases of prolonged administration (as with extended treatment of tuberculosis), are more likely to yield subtherapeutic levels in the gravid (or recently gravid) woman due to physiological alterations in drug distribution and clearance common to pregnancy.[19,20] Although the prototype quinolone antibiotic naladixic acid has been shown to cause cartilage damage and arthropathy in immature dogs and thus is relatively contraindicated for use in pregnancy,[21] the newer fluorinated compounds (e.g., ofloxicin, ciprofloxicin) are highly unlikely to have any important adverse fetal effects. For all of these reasons, however, these drugs should be avoided in the pregnant woman unless absolutely unreplaceable. On the other hand, it should be noted that the toxicities mentioned, especially after short treatment courses, are either minor or only theoretical. Therefore, accidental administration of any of these compounds to the pregnant woman with PID is not a major cause for alarm or consideration of a therapeutic abortion for fetal abnormalities. The obstetrician should merely discontinue the medication and substitute a more acceptable alternative.

Generally, antimicrobial drugs that have been considered appropriate for use in the pregnant woman include the penicillins, the cephalosporins, aztreonam (a monobactam antibiotic that may be substituted for the aminoglycosides), clindamycin, and erythromycin (which may occasionally be used intravenously in place of the tetracyclines as an antichlamydial drug). The physician should be able to organize an appropriate regimen for an individual patient out of these medications, taking into account hospital formulary restrictions, allergies, etc.

Conclusion

Pelvic inflammatory disease in the pregnant woman is an elusive diagnosis. This is true because, in the first instance, the diagnosis in patients presenting with fever, pain, and pregnancy may be confusing and often obscure. Second, and perhaps more confounding, is the bias of many obstetricians against its existence at all. Nevertheless, as a review of the literature indicates, PID and pelvic abscess do indeed complicate pregnancy and do so in unpredictable ways, contrary to what may be scientifically apparent. It remains an acute exercise of the medical art to make the appropriate diagnosis in such cases and escape with a viable pregnancy in the end.

For the physician who still has doubts about the existence of PID in pregnancy, it can only be underscored that this diagnosis must be entertained within the differential (i.e., Table 7.3), lest a potentially life-threatening disease be overlooked or treated improperly. At the very least, the physician can follow the strategy of considering PID in pregnancy a diagnosis of exclusion. It is correct to say that ruling out other entities on the list will greatly benefit the patient by leading her physician to the truth.

> *When you have eliminated the impossible,*
> *whatever remains, however improbable,*
> *must be the truth.*
>
> Sherlock Holmes
> *The Sign of the Four*

References

1. Novak E. (editorial comment) *Obstet Gynecol Surv* 1950;**5**:335–336.
2. Friedman S, Borrow ML. Pelvic inflammatory disease in pregnancy: A review of the literature and report of 5 cases. *Obstet Gynecol* 1959;**14**:417–425.
3. Lennon GG. Acute salpingitis during pregnancy. *J Obstet Gynecol Brit Emp* 1949;**56**:1035–1037.
4. McCord JM, Simmons CM. Acute purulent salpingitis during pregnancy. *Am J Obstet Gynecol* 1953;**65**:1136–1137.
5. Scott JM, Hay D. Acute salpingitis and pregnancy. *J Obstet Gynecol Brit Comm* 1954;**61**:788–792.
6. Lancet M, Cohen A. Acute purulent salpingitis in late pregnancy. *Obstet Gynecol* 1959;**14**:426–428.
7. Acosta AA, Mabray CR, Kaufman RH. Intrauterine pregnancy and coexistent pelvic inflammatory disease. *Obstet Gynecol* 1971;**37**:282–285.
8. Jafari K, Vilovic-Kos J, Webster A, Stepto RC. Tubo-ovarian abscess in pregnancy. *Acta Obstet Gynecol Scand* 1977;**56**:1–4.
9. Fuselier P, Alam A. Pregnancy complicated by pelvic abscess. *J Reprod Med* 1978;**21**:257–258.
10. Stubbs RE, Monif GRG. Ruptured tubo-ovarian abscess in pregnancy: Recovery of a penicillinase-producing strain of *Neisseria gonorrhoeae*. *Sex Transm Dis* 1985;**12**:235–237.
11. Davey MM, Guidozzi F. Ruptured tubo-ovarian abscess late in pregnancy. *S Afr Med J* 1987;**71**:120–121.
12. Blanchard AC, Pastorek JG, Weeks T. Pelvic inflammatory disease during pregnancy. *South Med J* 1987;**80**:1363–1365.
13. Andersen ES, Nielsen GL. The combination of pregnancy and acute salpingitis in a case of uterus didelphys. *Acta Obstet Gynecol Scand* 1988;**67**:175–176.

14. Kouyoumdjian A, Kirkpatrick J. Coexistence of an intrauterine pregnancy with both an ectopic pregnancy and salpingitis in the right fallopian tube: A case report. *J Reprod Med* 1990;**35**:824–826.

15. Metzger M. *Salpingitis et grossesse. Bull Soc Obstet Gynecol* (Paris) 1939; **28**:470–473.

16. Centers for Disease Control. Pelvic inflammatory disease: Guidelines for prevention and management. *MMWR* 1991;**40**(RR-5):17–21.

17. Expert Committee on Pelvic Inflammatory Disease. Pelvic inflammatory disease. Research directions in the 1990s. *Sex Transm Dis* 1991;**18**:46–64.

18. Hamod KA, Khouzami VA. Antibiotics in pregnancy, in Niebyl JR (ed): *Drug Use in Pregnancy*. Philadelphia, Lea & Febiger, 1982, pp 31–40.

19. Zaske DE, Cipolle RJ, Strate RG, et al. Rapid gentamicin elimination in obstetric patients. *Obstet Gynecol* 1980;**56**:559–564.

20. Pastorek JG, Ragan FA, Phelan M. Tobramycin dosing in the puerperal patient. *J Reprod Med* 1987;**32**:343–346.

21. Hooper DC, Wolfson JS. The fluoroquinolones: Pharmacology, clinical uses, and toxicities in humans. *Antimicrob Agents Chemother* 1985;**28**:716–721.

8
Pelvic Inflammatory Disease in the Adolescent Female

Vivien Igra, Jonathan Ellen, and Mary-Ann Shafer

Pelvic inflammatory disease (PID) is the most common serious complication of sexually transmitted diseases (STDs). Long-term sequelae of PID include ectopic pregnancy, chronic pelvic pain, and tubal infertility. Each year, over 1 million women experience an episode of PID, with approximately one-fifth of these cases occurring in adolescent females under 19 years of age.

Young women, in the second decade of life are at increased risk for PID compared to older women. Weström[1] estimated the risk of PID for a 15-year-old woman to be 10 times that of a 24-year-old woman. The combination of biological predisposition, behavioral risk factors, and cognitive immaturity that may limit an adolescent's ability to foresee potential consequences of their actions make the adolescent uniquely vulnerable to STDs, including PID. As a result, when controlled for rates of sexual activity, adolescents have the highest age-specific rates of PID. This chapter will discuss the epidemiology, risk factors, pathogenesis, clinical assessment, and management of PID in adolescent females including age-specific information when available.

Epidemiology

The majority of cases of acute PID are the result of ascending chlamydial and/or gonococcal endocervical infections. An estimated 3 million adolescents are infected with STDs each year in the United States.[2] The rate of gonococcal infection is three times higher for women aged 15 to 19 years than for any other age group. While the rates of gonococcal infection, among adults, declined between 1986 and 1989, the rate of decline among adolescents was the least among all age groups (see Figures 8.1 and 8.2). Rates of nonspecific urethritis (NSU), a proxy measure for rates of chlamydial infection in men, have been increasing since 1980 and are currently two to three times the rates of gonococcal urethritis. Among asymptomatic adolescent women, the prevalence of *Chlamydia trachomatis* isolated from the lower genital tract ranges from 8% to 40%, depending on the population characteristics.[3]

Approximately 10% to 17% of women with *N. gonorrhoeae* and 10% to 30% of women with *C. trachomatis* lower genital infections will develop PID.[4] The highest attack rate for PID occurs in sexually active adolescents less that 19 years of age.[5] From 1979 through 1988 an annual mean of 276,100 women were hospitalized for PID, 182,000 for acute PID, and the remainder for chronic PID.[6] Adolescents aged 15 to 19 years comprise 16% of those hospitalized with acute and chronic PID. Sexually active women in the younger adolescent age group have somewhat higher rates of hospitalization for acute PID and somewhat lower rates for chronic PID compared to older women.

Overall, hospitalization rates for acute PID declined for all age groups between 1979 and 1991 (see Figure 8.3). The relatively small decrease in hospitalization rates for 15- to 19-year-olds (10% compared with a 40% decrease for the 20- to 24-year-old group), resulted in the younger group's having the highest hospitalization rates for PID.[7] Hospitalization rates, however, do not necessarily accurately reflect disease rates as there has been a recent trend toward outpatient treatment for many medical conditions including PID. Regarding outpatient care, adolescents comprise 11% of the 350,000 office visits made for all types of PID in 1990.[2] Controlling for the approximately 50% of adolescent women who are not sexually active,

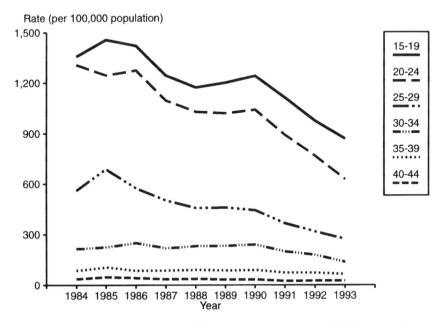

FIGURE 8.1. Gonorrhea—Age-specific rates among women 15–44 years of age, 1984–1993.

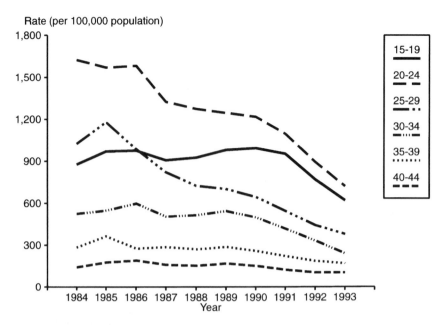

FIGURE 8.2. Gonorrhea—Age-specific rates among men 15–44 years of age, 1984–1993. Source: National Hospital Discharge Survey (National Center for Health Statistics, CDC).

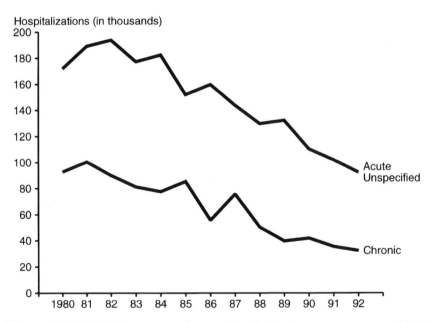

FIGURE 8.3. Pelvic inflammatory disease: Hospitalizations among women 15–44 years of age, United States, 1980–1992. Source: National Hospital Discharge Survey (National Center for Health Statistics, CDC).

the attack rates of PID become higher for 15- to 19-year-old women compared to all other age groups.

Risk Factors

Pelvic inflammatory disease is most commonly caused by *C. trachomatis* or *N. gonorrhoeae*. These organisms are primary pathogens of the endocervix and appear to cause PID by ascending to the upper genital tract. Therefore, factors that affect rates of chlamydial and gonococcal infection also affect rates of PID.

Behavioral Risk Factors

Behaviors including early sexual debut, multiple partners, and unprotected intercourse place adolescents at increased risk for STDs, including PID. The proportion of adolescent women, 15 to 19 years of age, engaging in sexual intercourse has increased steadily over the past 20 years, from 29% in 1970 to 52% in 1988. Approximately a third of this increase occurred in the 3 years from 1985 to 1988.[7] The largest increases were among the youngest adolescents.

Sexual activity among adolescents is often unplanned and sporadic. In addition, adolescents are at increased risk of exposure to STDs, because many of their relationships are nonmonogamous, or they may have numerous sexual partners over a short period of time (serial monogamy).[8] In 1988, adolescents who had sexual intercourse earlier in life reported greater numbers of sexual partners. Among 15- to 24-year-olds who initiated sexual intercourse before age 18, 75% reported having had two or more partners and 45% reported having had four or more partners. Among those who became sexually active after age 19, 20% reported having had more than one partner and only 1% had four or more partners.

Contraception

Younger adolescents are more likely to have multiple partners and are the least likely to use any form of contraception compared to older aged women. Among young women who had first intercourse before age 15 years, only 39% used any form of contraception, compared with 56% of those who delayed intercourse until they were aged 19 or older.[9] Among women aged 15 to 24 years, 46% reported using some contraceptive method at their most recent intercourse including 65% reporting birth control pill use, 21% condom use, 3% diaphragm use, and less than 1% IUD use.[10]

Barrier Contraception

The use of barrier contraceptives including condoms, diaphragms, and spermicide have been found to reduce risk of acquisition and transmission of STDs, including chlamydial and gonococcal infections and PID.[6] Keleghan[11] found that the diaphragm, with appropriate spermicide was most effective in reducing the risk of PID, followed by condoms used alone and spermicide used alone. Spermicide (Nonoxynol-9) used alone was least effective but combined with condom use was found to be as effective as the diaphragm used with spermicide. Barrier contraceptives have also been found to have a protective effect with respect to tubal infertility regardless of the history of PID.[12]

However, even though proven to be effective against STDs and PID, barrier contraceptive use by youth continues to be less than optimal. The use of diaphragms among female contraceptors aged 15 to 24 declined between 1982 and 1988 from 9% to 3%. While condom use among adolescent females appears to be increasing, only 21% of 15- to 24-year-old female contraceptors reported using a condom at their last intercourse.[10] Of young males 15–19 years of age in 1988, 56% reported using condoms at their most recent intercourse. Black male respondents had the highest reported rates of condom use at 66% followed by white male youth at 54% and Hispanic male youth at 53%.[13]

Oral Contraception

The role of oral contraceptives (OCs) in the development of PID is controversial. It appears that the effects of OCs vary with the stage of development of PID. For example, OCs appear to increase the risk of chlamydial endocervical infection, decrease the risk for symptomatic chlamydial PID (but not symptomatic gonococcal PID), and have no appreciable impact on tubal infertility.[14] Oral contraceptives may affect the course of PID by acting at different sites within the lower and upper genital tracts. For example, increased cervical ectropion appears to be the result of OC effects and chlamydia and specific types of gonococci attach preferentially to such tissue. In the upper tract, OCs may offer protection by decreasing the volume of menstrual blood available to potentiate bacterial growth and by providing the progestin-induced endocervical mucus thickening which impedes bacterial ascension from cervix to endometrium. When PID does develop in women using OCs, it appears to be less severe.[15] However, it is possible that while OCs decrease symptomatic PID rates, they have little effect on asymptomatic PID rates.

In conclusion OCs may increase the susceptibility to chlamydial lower genital tract infections but the role of OCs in the ascendence of *C. trachomatis* and *N. gonorrhoeae* to the upper genital tract remains unclear. If the effect of OCs is to reduce the risk of symptomatic PID, then the adolescent patient may be at greater risk for "silent PID," associated with ectopic pregnancy and infertility: adolescents and young adult women 15 to 24 years of age have high rates of STDs and OC use. The percent of contraceptors in this age group using OCs has increased steadily from 1982 to 1988 from 58% to 65%.[10] Because of the possible increased risk of "silent PID," adolescents using OCs should be routinely screened for STDs (see Prevention).

Intrauterine Device (IUD)

Intrauterine device use was reported by 3.4% of young female contraceptors age 15 to 24 years in 1982. This percentage declined to 0.2% in 1988.[10] A number of studies have demonstrated an increased risk of PID among women with IUDs.[16–18] Lee[16] found that those using the Dalkon Shield™ had five times the risk of PID compared to those using other types of IUDs. The risks use were greatest for younger women, never married women and those with multiple partners.[17] However, the Dalkon Sheild™ is no longer available in the United States. A recent review of studies evaluating available IUDs concluded that a significant increased risk for PID associated with IUD use was evident in the initial months following insertion.[19] Intrauterine devices also have been associated with an increased risk of tubal infertility[20] and ectopic pregnancy,[21] two of the most serious sequelae of PID.

In summary, it is recommended that the IUD not be prescribed for contraceptive use in young, nulliparous adolescent women especially those with a history of multiple sexual partners. Among monogamous, multiparous, older adolescent women, IUD use appears to carry minimal added risk for PID and may be a viable contraceptive alternative in selected cases.

Substance Use

High rates of alcohol, tobacco, and marijuana use among adolescents have been documented since the mid-1970s. In 1992, 17.5% of 12- to 19-year-olds reported at least one episode of heavy drinking (having five drinks or more in a row) in the prior month, 17.2% had used marijuana in the past, and 21.7% said they had smoked cigarettes within the last month.[22] A number of studies have linked substance use to early sexual debut.[24] In addition, alcohol and drug-induced sexual disinhibition is increasingly associated with failure to use condoms and multiple sexual partners, which places the adolescent female at increased risk for STDs and therefore PID.[8]

Ethnicity

Ethnicity should be considered a marker for STDs risk, rather than an active risk factor because it acts as a proxy for a combination of factors associated with acquisition of STDs such as socioeconomic status, access to health care, sexual partner networks, and behaviors. For example, black adolescents are more likely to be poor, more likely to initiate intercourse by age 16 and less likely to use condoms at their first intercourse than are white adolescents. Black adolescents have much higher rates of gonorrhea than their white counterparts. In addition, there may be a higher prevalence of STDs in black adolescent partner networks that contributes to their increased risk of infection. In King County, Washington in 1987, for example, the incidence of gonorrhea, among 15-year-old white women was 2,051/100,000 whereas the incidence among 15-year-old black women was 13,833/100,000, a sevenfold difference when adjusted for sexual experience.[25] Chlamydial rates have also been reported to be higher among black adolescents compared to white adolescents.[26]

A history of PID was reported by 3% of white and black adolescent females 15 to 19 years of age. However, black females 20 to 24 years of age reported a history of PID at twice the rate reported by white women the same age.[27] Ethnic differences by number of lifetime partners is also evident. A history of more than one lifetime male partner increased a black woman's risk of self-reported PID twofold and a white woman's risk increased by 30%.

Biological Risk Factors

Adolescent risk for STDs may be enhanced by pubertal changes. This biological predisposition is thought to be related to increased cervical ectopy and decreased immunological preparedness due to relatively lower exposure to potential pathogens compared to older women. In the prepubescent female, the ectocervix is covered in part by columnar epithelium. With progression through puberty, the columnar epithelium of the ectocervix recedes into the endocervix and is progressively replaced by squamous epithelium in adulthood (see Figure 8.4). The interface of the two types of cells is known as the "transition zone," the area of active cellular evolution is known as metaplasia, and combined these represent the zone of cervical ectopy. The columnar epithelium of the zone of ectopy are the preferential sites of attachment of *C. trachomatis* and some subtypes of *N. gonorrhoeae*.[28] As a result, factors that are associated with a more prominent zone of ectopy, including puberty and birth control pills, are also associated with an increased risk of these infections.

Hormonal changes that accompany puberty, result in an increasingly acidic vaginal milieu favoring the growth of normal acidophilic Doderlein bacteria.[29] During this transition, a younger adolescent may be more susceptible to potential pathogens that are associated with a less acidic vaginal environment; these include *Gardnerella vaginalis*, and anaerobes that are linked to bacterial vaginosis (BV). Recent findings have implicated BV as a risk factor itself for PID.[3]

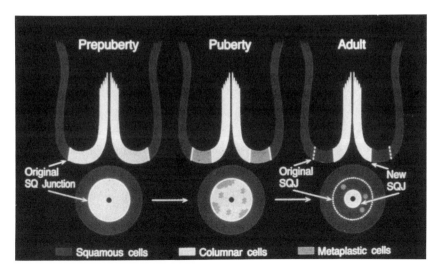

FIGURE 8.4. Cervical development.

Prior History of STDs or PID

Up to one-third of women with PID will experience a recurrence. Recurrences usually occur within 1 year of the initial infection and are less likely to be caused by *C. trachomatis* or *N. gonorrhoeae* than are the initial episodes.[1] In an analysis of self-reported PID,[27] a self-reported history of gonococcal, chlamydial, or herpes simplex infections increased the likelihood of PID by 2.5-fold. The relationship between prior STD or PID with a new episode of PID may be related to reinfection from untreated partners, inadequate therapy resulting in relapse of the first infection, increased vulnerability of damaged fallopian tubes, or the continued presence of risk factors such as younger age, multiple partners, or other biological or behavioral characteristics of the host that predisposed them to the initial infection.

Other Risk Factors for PID

Vaginal douching[30,31] and cigarette smoking[32,33] have been associated with an increased risk of PID. As a risk factor for STDs, substance use is also a risk factor for PID.[6] Operative procedures, such as dilatation and curettage, therapeutic abortion, tubal insufflation, and hysterosalpingography carry a relatively low risk for PID.

Microbial Etiology

As in adult women, most cases of PID among adolescents are caused by sexually transmitted organisms, *N. gonorrhoeae* or *C. trachomatis*. Other organisms implicated in the etiology of PID include *Mycoplasma hominis*,

Mycoplasma genitalium, *Ureaplasma urealyticum*, mixed anaerobic organisms (Bacteroides species and Peptostreptococci) and facultative bacteria (*Gardnerella vaginalis*, Streptococci, *E. coli*, and *H. influenza*).

The mycoplasmas, though recovered from the endocervix of women with PID, are rarely cultured from the upper genital tract and are most likely responsible for parametritis rather than true salpingitis.[34] The anaerobes and facultative agents may be present in normal postmenarchal vaginal flora and may predominate in BV. The role of BV in the etiology of PID remains unclear. Finally, certain viruses including human papillomavirus (HPV) and cytomegalovirus (CMV) have been isolated from the cervices of women with PID and may facilitate bacterial infection of the upper genital tract by disrupting the normal mechanical and immunological barriers to ascending infection to the upper genital tract.

Pathogenesis

Pelvic inflammatory disease is the result of ascension of lower genital infection from endocervix to the uterus and fallopian tubes, with a resulting inflammatory reaction in those structures. This ascent of the infectious agents may be hindered by insipated cervical mucus as with pregnancy or progestin-containing OCs. Conversely, ascent of pathogens may be facilitated by retrograde menstrual flow, transport by sperm, or by the presence of a conduit such as an IUD. As noted above, *N. gonorrhoeae* attaches preferentially to the cells of the transitional zone of the cervix, a prominent feature of the maturing adolescent. Chlamydia also attaches preferentially to the cells of the transition zone, which again increases the risk of PID in the adolescent.

Finally, the immune system has a potentially protective role with respect to the pathogenesis of PID. Antibodies such as secretory IgA, found in the mucosal secretions of the female genital tract interfere with attachment of pathogens to the cervical epithelium. Cellular immunity has also been found to play a role in combating bacterial and viral infections. It is possible that the immune system in the pubertal adolescent female is not fully mature and may not be as protective from PID compared to that of the adult female.

Diagnosis

Pelvic inflammatory disease is a clinical syndrome caused by ascending spread of microorganisms from the lower to the upper genital tract. The broad spectrum of syndromes that can be included under PID include endometritis, parametritis, salpingitis, oophoritis, pelvic peritonitis, and tub-ovarian abscess. A more narrow definition of PID refers to the clinical syndrome resulting from inflammation of the fallopian tubes or salpingitis. There are no uniformly accepted clinical criteria for the diagnosis of PID. Traditionally, laparoscopy has been considered the "gold standard" for the diagnosis of PID. However, laparoscopy is not feasible in most settings due to availability, cost, and potential risk to patients. For those reasons, clinical algorithms have been developed for the diagnosis of PID.

Most commonly used criteria are based on a classic Swedish series where women who presented with signs and symptoms of PID underwent laparoscopy for confirmation of their diagnosis. In that series, 65% were found to have salpingitis, 12% had other pelvic pathology, and 23% had normal pelvic findings. Utilizing the combination of signs and symptoms that distinguished the greatest number of affected individuals from the visually normal group, only 20% of the visually confirmed cases of salpingitis would have been detected.[35] Since that time, other clinical algorithms have been proposed.[34] However, a high degree of overlap has been found between confirmed salpingitis cases and visually normal cases at laparoscopy, irrespective of the clinical criteria used for diagnosis. In addition, mild or asymptomatic (silent) PID has been recognized as a major contributor to reproductive sequelae of PID.[36] As a result, the utility of algorithms dependent on a specific symptom complex has been questioned. Addition of microbiological, histopathological, and ultrasonographic criteria have been suggested to increase the accuracy of clinical diagnoses of PID.[6]

Clinical Presentation

The clinical presentation of PID varies from asymptomatic to life-threatening disease. Because the differential diagnosis for PID in the adolescent is extensive and includes surgical emergencies such as appendicitis, ectopic pregnancy, torsion of the ovary, and/or ovarian cyst as well as ruptured ovarian cysts, a direct approach to the history, including risk factors and symptoms, is critical.

History

Consent and Confidentiality

Every state has enacted laws permitting minors to consent for treatment of sexually transmitted diseases. Most states include a lower age limit, typically 12 or 14 at which a minor may consent to care. Most states that permit a minor to consent to care also permit the minor to control disclosure of information related to STD-related care. A few states permit, but do not require, the treating physician to notify the adolescents' parents.[37] Irrespective of such statutes, however, the health-care provider has an ethical obligation to inform the adolescent of the parameters of the minor's confidentiality prior to taking the history. Therefore, the approach to the history of an adolescent with suspected PID requires sensitivity and an awareness of the local statutes regarding consent and confidentiality when rendering STD care to minors. To facilitate open communication between the patient and the health-care provider, at least part of the history should be taken with the patient alone.

Sexual History

The adolescent patient may be reluctant to reveal her sexual activity if she perceives that there may be negative repercussions from her parents or her health-care provider. To obtain an accurate sexual history, the practitioner must provide the adolescent patient with privacy, confidentiality, and a sense of her own personal safety. The sexual history must include the patients age at sexual debut, the number of lifetime partners, the number of recent partners, and the patient's frequency of coitus. Further, it is important to ascertain the date of the most recent sexual encounter and what type of contraception, if any, was used. The patient should be questioned about the status of her partner(s), including her partner's sexual history and possible exposure or symptoms of an STD.

Menstrual History

A detailed menstrual history is particularly important to elicit in the adolescent patient. Irregular bleeding may be a sign of a maturing hypothalamic–pituitary–gonadal axis within the first 12 to 24 months after menarche or a sign of possible upper genital tract infection as is found in adult women. The onset of normal physiological dysmenorrhea usually parallels the onset of ovulatory cycles in adolescents. For this reason, it may be more difficult for the clinician to differentiate physiological from pathological dysmenorrhea when the adolescent presents with dysmenorrhea for the first time. The menstrual history includes the patient's age at menarche, the date of her most recent menses, and whether or not it was atypical in duration or intensity. The frequency of vaginal bleeding and any history of unusual dysmenorrhea should also be elicited.

Irregular bleeding is associated with endometritis and salpingitis. In one study of laparoscopically confirmed PID, irregular bleeding was significantly more common among those with chlamydial PID than in nonchlamydial disease.[38] Amenorrhea may be a sign of pregnancy, intrauterine or ectopic. Menorrhagia may indicate a spontaneous complete or incomplete abortion. Onset of symptoms of gonococcal and chlamydial salpingitis occurs most often within 7 days of menses.[39] This is thought to be related to the loss of the mucus plug with subsequent predisposition to ascending infection. Nongonococcal facultative aerobes and anaerobes, however, are found to cause salpingitis equally throughout the menstrual cycle.

Contraceptive History

When obtaining a contraceptive history from an adolescent, it is important to ascertain the type of contraception used, and that the method was used correctly and consistently. For example, condoms may be used with casual partners but not with "main" partners. Birth control pills may have been missed or taken sporadically. If the adolescent is using an IUD, the type of IUD and the date of insertion should be elicited because a higher incidence of PID has been noted within the 4 weeks following insertion of certain types of IUDs (See IUD discussion above).

Other History

As mentioned above, a prior history of STDs or PID increases the current risk for PID. Any history of urogenital or pelvic operative procedures such as IUD placement, therapeutic abortion, or hysterosalpingography should alert the practitioner to the possibility of PID.

Symptoms

Many of the symptoms associated with PID (see Table 8.1) appear to be as common with laparoscopically proven salpingitis as with normal pelvic findings.[35] Increasing the number of clinical criteria required for a diagnosis of PID increased the specificity but only at a cost to the sensitivity. In other words, the more clinical criteria required to make a diagnosis of PID, the greater the risk of missing less symptomatic cases of salpingitis.

Pain

Abdominal pain associated with PID is usually located in the lower quadrants and is often bilateral. Right-upper quadrant pain, reported by ~5% of women with PID, suggests perihepatitis that can accompany chlamydial or gonococcal PID.[1] Golden and others,[5] found that among adolescents with PID, gonococcal disease was associated with a shorter duration of pain prior to presentation than was chlamydial disease (3 days vs. 6 days $p < 0.05$). Abdominal pain was once considered the sine qua non of PID. However, more recently the importance of asymptomatic PID has come to be appreciated. In one study, endometritis was found in 40% of women with cervicitis with no symptoms of PID.[40] Subclinical, asymptomatic silent PID has been linked to adverse reproductive sequelae including ectopic pregnancy and tubal infertility. More than one-half of

TABLE 8.1. Differential diagnoses of PID in the adolescent female by system.

Location	Diagnoses
Reproductive tract	Ectopic pregnancy
	Intrauterine pregnancy
	Dysmenorrhea
	Endometriosis
	Ruptured corpus luteum cyst
	Spontaneous abortion
	Torsion of the ovary
Urinary tract	Cystitis
	Pyelonephritis
	Ureteral calculi
	Urethritis
Gastrointestinal tract	Appendicitis
	Diverticulitis
	Cholecystitis
	Gastroenteritis
	Hepatitis
	Inflammatory bowel disease
Other	Pleuritis
	Pneumonia
	Sickle cell crisis
	Trauma

women with documented tubal occlusion report no history of PID despite serological evidence of past chlamydial infection. As a result, the most recent criteria suggested by the CDC do not require the presence of abdominal pain for the diagnosis of PID.[6]

Other painful symptoms associated with PID include dysmenorrhea, dyspareunia, and dysuria. Reported pelvic pain with intercourse may be related to cervical motion tenderness, a sign of PID. Dysuria may indicate concurrent urethral infection with chlamydia, gonococci, or mycoplasmas[1] or other urinary tract diseases.

Finally, it is particularly important to recognize the difficulty of assessing the location, degree, and pathogenesis of abdominal pain in a fearful adolescent female who is inexperienced with gynecological examinations. Clinical errors can be made if a complaint from an adolescent is too readily dismissed as insignificant.

Fever

Although fever was reported in less than one-half of subjects with laparoscopically verified PID, this symptom was twice as common among cases of salpingitis than in the "visually normal" group $p < 0.001$.[35] Similar to findings in adult women,[41] adolescents with gonococcal PID have been found to have higher mean maximum temperatures than adolescents with chlamydial-associated PID.[5]

Gastrointestinal Symptoms

While nausea and vomiting may be seen in as many as 10% of cases of PID,[35] they occur more frequently with gastrointestinal pathology such as appendicitis. A more complete discussion of symptoms is found elsewhere in this text.

Physical Assessment

The physical assessment of a patient with suspected PID must include an abdominal, vaginal, speculum, and bimanual pelvic examination. For some adolescents presenting with symptoms consistent with PID, this may be the first pelvic examination. In an adolescent who is frightened of the procedure and of possible disclosure of her sexual activity, it is often difficult to differentiate pain and anxiety related to the pelvic examination itself from pain secondary to pelvic pathology. When assessing the adolescent patient, and experienced clinician should perform the examination when possible. It is important to assist the adolescent in decreasing her anxiety about the exam by gently explaining procedures throughout the examination. A negative experience with an initial pelvic examination may discourage health-seeking behavior in the future.

Abdominal Tenderness

Lower abdominal tenderness, bilateral adnexal tenderness, and cervical motion tenderness are the minimum criteria, suggested by the CDC for the clinical diagnosis of PID.[6] Uterine tenderness is suggestive of endometritis. Palpation of an adnexal mass may suggest a tubo-ovarian abscess or tubal pregnancy.

Vaginal Discharge

The presence of a foul smelling vaginal discharge may suggest BV. In this syndrome, lactobacilli are, in part, replaced by *Gardnerella vaginalis*, anaerobic streptococci, bacteroides species or genital mycoplasmas. Bacterial vaginosis has been linked to polymicrobial PID.[28]

Cervical Discharge

As with adult women, a mucopurulent discharge noted on a white-tipped swab from the cervical os may be a sign of chlamydial or gonococcal cervicitis, endometritis, or salpingitis in the adolescent.[42] The gram-stained specimen on a slide with greater than 30 white blood cells/oil emersion field is correlated with mucopurulent cervicitis, chlamydial, or gonococcal infection.[43] A gram stain, reviewed by an experienced professional, may also reveal intracellular diplococci, which may be consistent with gonococcal infection.

Laboratory Evaluation

Laboratory tests recommended for all suspected cases of PID include: (1) cervical cultures for *N. gonorrhoeae* and (2) cervical culture or nonculture test for *C. trachomatis*.[6] Among adolescents with PID, endocervical *N. gonorrhoeae* was detected in 36% and *C. trachomatis* in 45% of patients examined.[5] Tissue culture has been the gold standard for the diagnosis of chlamydial infection. This is expensive, requires somewhat sophisticated laboratory techniques, and is not always available at the time of the evaluation of PID. As a result, a number of nonculture tests for chlamydia have been developed that are rapid, less expensive, and require less technical expertise. These include direct monofluorescent antibody for the detection of antigen and chlamydial enzyme linked immunoassay. A more complete discussion of laboratory testing for PID may be found elsewhere in this text.

Pregnancy Test

A sensitive urine or serum pregnancy test is imperative to rule out possible ectopic or intrauterine pregnancy before the diagnosis of PID is made and definitive treatment begun in the adolescent patient.

Adjunctive Procedures

A more elaborate diagnostic evaluation may be warranted to eliminate the possibilities of surgical emergencies such as ectopic pregnancy, ruptured ovarian cysts, tubo-ovarian abscess (TOA), or appendicitis. When the diagnosis of PID is in doubt or if the patient does not appear to be responding to conventional therapy for PID, further diagnostic evaluation is necessary.

Ultrasound has been used successfully in adolescents to detect clinically unsuspected tubo-ovarian abscesses[44] and to rule out selected competing diagnoses in adolescents that would require surgical intervention.[45] More recently, intravaginal ultrasonography has been used in patients with suspected PID as an alternative to laparoscopy and an adjunct to endometrial biopsy.[36,46] While potentially promising techniques are refined, the value of ultrasound in early or mild PID, in the absence of anatomic distortion has yet to be delineated. Laparoscopy with or without fimbrial biopsy, culdocentesis (to determine the presence of purulent material from the cul de sac), and endometrial biopsy (which provides histopathological evidence of disease) are used as adjunctive procedures when the diagnosis of PID is uncertain and the techniques are available. However, in most cases, such procedures are unwarranted, expensive, and carry risk to the patient. A more comprehensive discussion of these procedures is found elsewhere in this text.

Differential Diagnosis

The differential diagnosis of PID in adolescents is extensive. It is important to eliminate competing diagnoses that could be life-threatening or require immediate surgical intervention. In particular, an evaluation for intrauterine and ectopic pregnancy can be accomplished with a sensitive urine or serological pregnancy test. Common differential diagnoses for PID in the adolescent female can be found in Table 8.1.

Management

Hospitalization

Hospitalization of adolescents with PID is advocated to eliminate compliance issues and to minimize possible complications resulting in long-term sequelae including ectopic pregnancy, infertility, and chronic pelvic pain.

Antibiotic Therapy

Currently recommended antimicrobial regimens for the treatment of PID are broad spectrum because no single agent has proven effective against *C. trachomatis*, *N. gonorrhoeae*, anaerobes, gram-negative rods, and streptococci. The current CDC recommendations for inpatient treatment of PID include combinations of antibiotics: Either (1) β-lactam with doxycycline or (2) clindamycin with an aminoglycocide (see Table 8.2 below). Once antibiotics have been instituted, careful follow up is critical. If the patient's symptoms and signs worsen or do not improve within 48 to 72 h of onset of therapy, a complete reevaluation of the diagnosis and treatment plan is necessary including a pelvic examination. Other diagnoses to consider include tubo-ovarian abscess, appendicitis, ruptured ovarian cyst or adnexal torsion. Complicated PID may require more prolonged hospitalization and rarely, surgical intervention (see below). In addition, there are some early indications that human immunodeficiency virus (HIV) infected women

TABLE 8.2. Inpatient therapy for PID (CDC 1993).

Regimen A	Regimen B
Cefoxitin 2 g i.v. every 6 h or cefotetan 2 g i.v. every 12 h	Clindamycin 900 mg i.v. every 8 h
PLUS	PLUS
Doxycycline 100 mg p.o. or i.v. every 12 h	Gentamicin 2 mg/kg loading dose i.m. or i.v. followed by a maintenance dose of 1.5 mg/kg i.v. every 8 h

with PID may be at increased risk for more severe disease and may be more likely to require operative intervention. This will have increasing relevance for adolescent PID patients as rates of HIV infection among adolescent females continue to rise with current figures as high as 4.2% in some populations.[47]

Complications

Tubo-ovarian Abscess

In a study of adolescents with PID, Golden[5] found that 20% developed TOAs. Comparable rates are found among older women with PID. The diagnosis of TOA is made when a palpable mass is defined in the adnexa in the context of PID. The clinical diagnosis of TOA is notoriously unreliable. For example among adolescents with PID, Golden and others[5] found that, fewer than one-third of those who subsequently had a TOA confirmed by ultrasound were initially suspected clinically. As a result of the difficulty in accurately determining the presence of a TOA in PID, liberal use of ultrasound has been advocated to investigate suspected TOA among adolescents. Antimicrobial therapy for TOA requires adequate coverage against resistant gram-negative anaerobes particularly bacteroides species. Clindamycin and metronidazole are considered among the most effective agents for the treatment of TOAs. Parenteral broad spectrum β-lactam agents, combined with oral doxycycline also appear to be as effective as clindamycin containing regimens for the treatment of TOA.[48] Surgical intervention should be considered in the event of antibiotic failure, that is, clinical deterioration or increase in the size of the abscess. Because the adolescent female has clearly not completed her reproductive life, it is imperative to preserve as much reproductive function as possible when surgery is required for PID in this age group.

Perihepatitis

The Fitz–Hugh–Curtis Syndrome (FHCS) or perihepatitis, occurs in 15% to 30% of women with PID and involves inflammation of the capsule of the liver associated with salpingitis. Classically, it consists of "violin string"

adhesions between the liver capsule and the diaphragm or anterior peritoneal surface. Early studies found that perihepatitis was associated with
gonococcal infection. More recently chlamydial infection, which is common
among adolescents, has been found to predominate.[49]

Long-Term Sequelae

One-fourth of all women who have had acute PID will experience one or
more long-term sequelae.[34] Long-term sequelae of PID, including ectopic
pregnancy and tubal infertility, are related to damage to the fallopian tubes.
Damage may include loss of ciliary motility of the tubal mucosa, narrowing
or occlusion of the tubal lumen from scarring or adhesions, or the formation
of microscopic blind pockets in the mucosa.

Ectopic Pregnancy

The incidence of ectopic pregnancy has increased fivefold in the past 20
years and is the leading cause of death in the first trimester of pregnancy.[50]
Twenty to 40% of women who have an ectopic pregnancy will not be able
to conceive again and 20% will have a second ectopic pregnancy.[21] Rates
of ectopic pregnancy among adolescents are lower than those among older
women. However, the death rate for adolescents from ectopic pregnancy is
substantially higher than for older age groups. The death rate for ectopic
pregnancy among nonwhite adolescents is five times the rate for white teens
in the United States.[51] This increased mortality rate in this age group may be
due to a delay in seeking treatment by the adolescent because of fear or
ignorance regarding intrauterine and ectopic pregnancy. In addition, when
a history of sexual activity is not forthcoming from the young patient, the
possibility of ectopic pregnancy may not be recognized by the clinician.

The diagnosis of ectopic pregnancy should be suspected in any sexually
active adolescent female who presents with a history of lower abdominal
pain, amenorrhea, and/or irregular vaginal bleeding. The history and physical assessment parallel that for PID. The adolescent may be unaware of
her pregnancy or unwilling to disclose sexual activity. In one series, 71%
of adolescents diagnosed with tubal pregnancy denied knowing that they
were pregnant prior to presenting to the emergency room.[52] Therefore, it is
important for the clinician to consider ectopic pregnancy in any postmenarchal adolescent female who presents with unexplained abdominal pain.

Infertility and Other Sequelae

In addition to ectopic pregnancy, another potential tragedy resulting from
PID for the adolescent is the development of infertility before she desires to
become pregnant. One in 12 women of child-bearing age has impaired
ability to have children. Involuntary infertility occurs in 20% of women

after at least one episode of PID and is most likely the result of damage to fallopian tubes.[34] The incidence of tubal occlusion increases with the number of episodes of PID. Among women 15 to 24 years of age, infertility rates are 9% after the first infection, 27% after the second, and 52% after three or more infections.[1] Silent or asymptomatic PID related to C. trachomatis infection may play a significant role in the genesis of tubal infertility. Other important sequelae of PID include chronic pelvic pain, dyspareunia, pelvic adhesions, and increased risk for recurrent PID. Such sequelae are particularly important to adolescents who potentially have long reproductive lives ahead.

Prevention

PID prevention can be divided into the following strategies: primary prevention to reduce exposure to STDs, secondary prevention to enhance early recognition and appropriate treatment of STDs to reduce the incidence of PID and tertiary prevention, and to detect and treat PID in a timely manner to prevent short- and long-term sequelae. The most important of these, for adolescents, is primary prevention.

Effective primary prevention of PID and other STDs requires a multidimensional approach that is beyond the scope of this chapter. The CDC has recommended community health promotion and education, including school-based programs and the media to inform adolescents about how to reduce their risk for STDs.[6] Primary prevention, for the medical practitioner, begins with assessment of risk for STDs. Any factor that places an adolescent at risk for STD, increases their risk for PID. Risk factors for STDs have been elaborated above. Essentially all sexually active adolescents are at risk for STDs. There is a substantial role, however, for education involving risk reduction for this group. Those adolescents who are not engaging in sexual activity should be encouraged to postpone initiating coitus as younger adolescents are at greater risk for STDs and PID. Adolescents who are sexually active should be encouraged to limit their number of partners and to use barrier contraception consistently.

Education must include the role of substance use in the transmission of STDs. Adolescents need to understand that the impaired judgement that accompanies substance use may lead to unplanned intercourse with inadequate protection against STDs and pregnancy. Educational efforts involving adolescents that incorporate skills training have been found to be more effective than those that are solely information-based.[8] Examples of skill-building include learning to use a condom or role-playing sexual decision-making during an office visit or school program. Finally, adolescent need to be educated about STD symptoms and to be encouraged to seek medical attention if these symptoms occur or in the event of unprotected intercourse.

Secondary prevention involves detecting and treating STDs. A number of studies have attempted to use epidemiological evidence to develop screening protocols for sexually transmitted diseases. A recent study found that age less than 25 years was by far the best predictor of the presence of chlamydial infection.[53] No other symptom, behavior, or demographic characteristic reliably predicted infection. This study and others point to the need for routine STD screening for all sexually active adolescents. Screening for STDs is particularly important before procedures such as therapeutic abortions or IUD insertions. These procedures have been associated with PID through iatrogenic spread of lower genital tract infections. When an STD is suspected, prompt treatment using the most recent CDC guidelines should ensue, even before confirmatory tests are available. Delay in treatment, such as waiting for confirmation of the diagnosis, could result in ascension of the infection with development of PID as well as unnecessary spread of the STD. In addition, partners must be aggressively sought, screened, and treated or referred for treatment. A test of cure should be performed 2 weeks after completing treatment for chlancydial infections. This follow-up visit can be utilized to reinforce risk reduction education.

Tertiary prevention requires early recognition and adequate treatment of PID to mitigate the sequelae. Hospitalization is recommended for all adolescents. A test of cure should be performed 2 weeks after treatment has been completed, and partners must be treated as well. Adolescents with a history of PID are at risk for recurrence and late sequelae and should be followed on a regular basis with pelvic examinations and STD screening tests as indicated. In summary, in order to prevent PID and its sequelae, adolescents must be educated about STD transmission, advised to use barrier contraception consistently, routinely screened and treated appropriately for STDs and their sexual partners should be treated or referred for treatment as needed.

Conclusion

Pelvic inflammatory disease is an important complication of STDs in adolescent women. Adolescent women may be more susceptible to upper genital tract infection than older women due to their unique biological predisposition and sexual behaviors. In addition, because adolescent women are just beginning their reproductive lives, they are at the greatest risk for reproductive health problems resulting from delayed or missed diagnosis of PID. As a result, it is imperative to consider PID in the differential diagnosis for all young women who present with abdominal pain.

References

1. Weström L, Mardh P-A. Acute pelvic inflammatory disease (PID), in Mardh P-A, Sparling PF, Wiesner PJ, Holmes KK (eds): *Sexually Transmitted Diseases*. New York, McGraw-Hill Information Services Co., 1990, pp 593–613.

2. Centers for Disease Control. Sexually transmitted disease surveillance 1992. U.S. Department of Health and Human Services, Public Health Service 1993.

3. Cates W, Rolfs RT, Aral SO. Sexually transmitted diseases, pelvic inflammatory disease, and infertility: An epidemiologic update. *Epidemiol Rev* 1990;**12**: 199–220.

4. Washington AE, Sweet RL, Shafer MA. Pelvic inflammatory disease and its sequelae in adolescents. *J Adolesc Health Care* 1985;**6**:298–310.

5. Golden N, Neuhoff S, Cohen H. Pelvic inflammatory disease in adolescents. *J Pediatr* 1989;**114**:138–143.

6. Centers for Disease Control. Pelvic inflammatory disease: Guidelines for prevention and management. *MMWR* 1991;**40**(no.RR-5):1–25.

7. Centers for Disease Control. Premarital sexual experience among adolescent women—United States, 1970–88. *MMWR* 1991;**39**(51,52):929–932.

8. Boyer CB. Psychosocial, behavioral and educational factors in preventing sexually transmitted diseases, in Schydlower M, and Shafer M-A (eds): *AIDS and Other Sexually Transmitted Diseases. Adolescent Medicine: State of the Arts Review*, Philadelphia: Hanley & Belfus, Inc., 1990, pp 597–613.

9. Mosher WD, McNally JW. Contraceptive use at first premarital intercourse: United States, 1965–1988. *Fam Plann Perspect* 1991;**23**:108–128.

10. Centers for Disease Control. Contraceptive use in the United States, 1973–88. *Advance Data* 1990;182.

11. Kelaghan J, Rubin GL, Ory HW, Layde PM. Barrier-method contraceptives and pelvic inflammatory disease. *JAMA* 1982;**248**:184–187.

12. Cramer DW, Goldman MB, Schiff I, Belisle S, Albrecht B, Stadel B, Gibson M, Wilson E, Stillman R, Thompson I. The relationship of tubal infertility to barrier method and oral contraceptive use. *JAMA* 1987;**257**:2446–2450.

13. Sonenstein FL, Pleck JH, and Ku, LC. Sexual activity, condoms use, and AIDS awareness among adolescent males. *Fam. Plan. Perspectives*, 1989;**21**(4): 152–158.

14. Washington AE, Katz P. Cost of and payment source for pelvic inflammatory disease: Trends and projections, 1983 through 2000. *JAMA* 1991;**266**: 2565–2569.

15. Rice PA, Schachter J. Pathogenesis of pelvic inflammatory disease: What are the questions? *JAMA* 1991;**266**:2587–2593.

16. Lee NC, Rubin GL, Borucki R. The intrauterine device and pelvic inflammatory disease revisited: New results from the Women's Health Study. *Obstet Gynecol* 1988;**72**:1–6.

17. Lee NC, Rubin GL, Ory HW, Burkman RT. Type of intrauterine device and the risk of pelvic inflammatory disease. *Obstet Gynecol* 1983;**62**:1–6.

18. Kaufman DW, Watson J, Rosenberg L, Helmrich SP, Miller DR, Miettinen OS, Stolley PD, Shapiro S. The effect of different types of intrauterine devices on the risk of pelvic inflammatory disease. *JAMA* 1983;**250**:759–762.

19. Kessel E. Pelvic inflammatory disease with intrauterine device use: A reassessment. *Fertil Steril* 1989;**51**:1–11.

20. Cramer DW, Schiff I, Schoenbaum SC, Gibson M, Belisle S, Albrecht B, Stillman RJ, Berger MJ, Wilson E, Stadel BV, et al. Tubal infertility and the intrauterine device. *N Engl J Med* 1985;**312**:941–947.

21. Chow WH, Daling JR, Cates W Jr, Greenberg RS. Epidemiology of ectopic pregnancy. *Epidemiol Rev* 1987;**9**:70–94.

22. Centers for Disease Control. Health behaviors among adolescents who do and do not attend school—United States, 1992. *MMWR* 1994;**43**:129–132.

23. Mott FL, Haurin RJ. Linkages between sexual activity and alcohol and drug use among American adolescents. *Fam Plann Perspect* 1988;**20**:128–136.

24. Kandel DB, Raveis VH. Cessation of illicit drug use in young adulthood. *Arch Gen Psychiatry* 1989;**46**:109–116.

25. Rice RJ, Roberts PL, Handsfield HH, Holmes KK. Sociodemographic distribution of gonorrhea incidence: Implications for prevention and behavioral research. *Am J Public Health* 1991;**81**:1252–1258.

26. Shafer M-A, Beck A, Blain B. *Chlamydia trachomatis*: Important relationships to race, contraception, lower genital tract, and Papanicolaou smears. *J Pediatr* 1984;**104**:141.

27. Aral SG, Mosher WD, Cates W. Self-reported pelvic inflammatory disease in the United States, 1988. *JAMA* 1991;**266**:2570–2573.

28. National Institutes of Health. Pelvic inflammatory disease. *Sex Transm Dis* 1991;**1**:46–64.

29. Shafer M-A, Sweet RL. Pelvic inflammatory disease in adolescent females, in Schydlower M, Shafer M-A (eds): *AIDS and Other Sexually Transmitted Diseases. Adolescent Medicine: State of the Art Reviews*. Philadelphia, Hanley & Belfus, Inc., 1990.

30. Forrest KA, Washington AE, Daling JR, Sweet RL. Vaginal douching as a possible risk factor for pelvic inflammatory disease. *J Natl Med Assoc* 1989;**81**:159–165.

31. Wølner-Hanssen P, Eschenbach DA, Paavonen J, Stevens CE, Kiviat N, Critchlow C, DeRouen T, Koutsky L, Holmes KK. Association between vaginal douching and acute pelvic inflammatory disease. *JAMA* 1990;**263**:1936–1941.

32. Scholes D, Daling JR, Stergachis AS. Current cigarette smoking and risk of acute pelvic inflammatory disease. *AJPH* 1992;**82**:1252–1355.

33. Marchbanks PA, Lee NC, Peterson HB. Cigarette smoking as a risk factor for pelvic inflammatory disease. *Am J Obstet Gynecol* 1990;**162**:639–644.

34. Sweet RL, Schachter J, Robbie MO. Failure of beta-lactam antibiotics to eradicate *Chlamydia trachomatis* in the endometrium despite apparent clinical cure of acute salpingitis. *JAMA* 1983;**250**:2641–2645.

35. Jacobson L, Weström L. Objectivized diagnosis of acute pelvic inflammatory disease. *Am J Obstet Gynecol* 1969;**105**:1088–1098.

36. Wølner-Hanssen P, Kiviat NB, Holmes KK. Atypical pelvic inflammatory disease: Subacute, chronic, or subclinical upper genital tract infection in women, in Mardh P-A, Sparling PF, Wiesner PJ, Holmes KK (eds): *Sexually Transmitted Diseases*. New York, McGraw-Hill Information Services Co., 1990, pp 615–620.

37. English A. Treating adolescents: Legal and ethical considerations. *Medical Clin North Am* 1990;**74**:1097–1113.

38. Svensson L, Weström L, Ripa KT, Mardh P-A. Differences in some clinical and laboratory parameters in acute salpingitis related to culture and serologic findings. *Am J Obstet Gynecol* 1980;**138**:1017–1021.

39. Sweet RL, Blankfort-Doyle M, Robbie MO, Schachter J. The occurrence of chlamydial and gonococcal salpingitis during the menstrual cycle. *JAMA* 1986;**255**:2062–2064.

40. Paavonen J, Kiviat N, Brunham RC, Stevens CE, Kuo CC, Stamm WE, Miettinen A, Soules M, Eschenbach DA, Holmes KK. Prevalence and manifes-

tations of endometritis among women with cervicitis. *Am J Obstet Gynecol* 1985;**152**:280–286.

41. Weström L, Mardh P-A. Chlamydial salpingitis. *Br Med Bull* 1983;**39**:145–150.
42. Moscicki AB, Winkler B, Irwin CE Jr, Schachter J. Differences in biologic maturation, sexual behavior, and sexually transmitted disease between adolescents with and without cervical intraepithelial neoplasia. *J Pediatr* 1989;**115**: 487–493.
43. Soper D. Diagnosis and laparoscopic grading of acute salpingitis. *Am J Obstet Gynecol* 1991;**164**:1370–1376.
44. Golden N, Cohen H, Gennari G, Neuhoff S. The use of pelvic ultrasonography in the evaluation of adolescents with pelvic inflammatory disease. *AJDC* 1987;**141**:1235–1238.
45. Risser WL, Pokorny SF, Maklad NF. Ultrasound examination of adolescent females with lower abdominal pain. *J Adolesc Health Care* 1988;**9**:407–410.
46. Cacciatore B, Leminen A, Ingman-Friberg S, Ylostalo P, Paavonen J. Transvaginal sonographic findings in ambulatory patients with suspected pelvic inflammatory disease. *Obstet Gynecol* 1992;**80**:912–916.
47. Stricof RL, Kennedy JT, Nattell TC, Weisfuse IB, Novick LF. HIV seroprevalence in a facility for runaway and homeless adolescents. *Am J Public Health* 1991;**81**:50s–53s.
48. Reed SD, Landers DV, Sweet RL. Antibiotic treatment of tuboovarian abscess: Comparison of broad-spectrum beta-lactam agents versus clindamycin-containing regimens. *Am J Obstet Gynecol* 1991;**164**:1556–1562.
49. Lopez-Zeno JA, Keith LG, Berger GS. The Fitz-Hugh-Curtis syndrome revisited. Changing perspectives after half a century. *J Reprod Med* 1985;**30**:567–582.
50. Ammerman S, Shafer M-A, Snyder D. Ectopic pregnancy in adolescents: a clinical review for pediatricians. *J Pediatr* 1990;**117**:677–686.
51. Centers for Disease Control. Ectopic pregnancy surveillance, United States, 1970–1987. *MMWR* 1997;**39**(SS-4):9–17.
52. Gale CL, Stovall TG, Muram D. Tubal pregnancy in adolescence. *J Adolesc Health Care* 1990;**11**:485–489.
53. Winter L, Goldy AS, Baer C. Prevalence and epidemiologic correlates of Chlamydia trachomatis in rural and urban populations. *Sex Transm Dis* 1990;**17**:30–36.

9
Pelvic Inflammatory Disease and HIV-1 Infection

Abner P. Korn and Daniel V. Landers

It is no surprise that women with pelvic inflammatory disease (PID) have a significantly higher prevalence of human immunodeficiency virus (HIV) seropositivity than women without such a history. Pelvic inflammatory disease and sexually acquired HIV infection have many common risk factors. There has also been concern that because HIV infection can lead to altered immune function, the acute infection and subsequent sequelae of PID may be worse in HIV-infected women. The Centers for Disease Control, included PID, particularly if complicated by tubo-ovarian abscess, as a category B condition in their 1993 revised classification system for HIV infection.[1] This category includes clinical conditions attributable to HIV infection or indicative of a defect in cell-mediated immunity or conditions considered to have a clinical course complicated by HIV.

There are differing opinions as to whether the clinical course of PID is altered in HIV-infected women. It has been suggested that PID may occur more frequently in HIV+ women colonized with *Neisseria gonorrhoeae* and/or *Chlamydia trachomatis* especially in the presence of low CD4 cell counts. The clinical presentation and the response to treatment may also be affected in HIV+ women particularly in those with severe immunocompromise. In addition, there are other confounding variables that may influence the course of PID in HIV-infected individuals. Bacterial vaginosis (BV) occurs more frequently in HIV+ women than in uninfected women and has been identified as a risk factor for developing PID.[2] Behavioral factors may also influence the course of PID in HIV+ women. For example, HIV-infected injection drug users (IDU) often obtain medical care later and less often than nondrug users. More severe presentations of PID can be expected if there is a delay in seeking medical attention. These theoretical concerns have yet to be addressed in large studies of HIV-infected women.

This chapter focuses on the current knowledge of PID and HIV based on the relatively limited data available at the present time. Particular attention is paid to the potential influences of HIV infection on the presentation, clinical course, and response to therapy seen in HIV-infected women with PID.

Risk Factors and Prevalence

Confection with sexually transmitted organisms is a common occurrence likely related to common risk factors. The risk of becoming infected with *N. gonorrhoeae* or *C. trachomatis*, the organisms frequently responsible for PID, is enhanced or diminished by the same factors affecting HIV transmission. The transmission of HIV, gonorrhea, and chlamydia are all reduced by the use of barrier contraceptives such as condoms.[3] Conversely, women with multiple sexual contacts who do not use barrier contraception are at an increased risk for both HIV and PID.

Infection with numerous other sexually transmitted organisms increases the risk of HIV acquisition. This includes the sexually transmitted organisms producing ulceration in the lower genital tract such as *T. palladum* and *H. ducreyi* and many of the nonulcerative sexually transmitted organisms including *C. trachomatis* and *Trichomonas vaginalis*.[2,4] An increased risk of sexual acquisition of HIV has also been associated with BV.[2,5]

A higher prevalence of many sexually transmitted organisms has been reported in a number of HIV+ cohorts when compared to HIV− controls. In a New York City cohort, *N. gonorrhoeae* was isolated from 38% and salpingitis diagnosed in 33% of HIV+ adolescents.[6] In another report, trichomonas was found in 26.9%, syphilis in 22.2%, herpes simplex virus in 17.8%, *C. trachomatis* in 12.3%. *N. gonorrhoeae* in 7.2%, and PID in 5.3% of 224 HIV+ women followed in Louisiana from 1987 to 1991 (mean duration of follow-up was 18 months).[7]

The reported seroprevalence of HIV infection in women with acute PID ranges from 2.7% to 22%[8-15] (Table 9.1). HIV testing in women diagnosed with PID is clearly warranted given these data regarding HIV prevalence in women with PID.

TABLE 9.1. The reported seroprevalence of HIV infection in women with acute PID.

Location	Seroprevalence (%)	Last year of study
Baragwanath Hospital[8]	2.7 (21/772)	1990
San Francisco General Hospital[9]	6.7 (8/119)	1988
Gweru Provincial Hospital, Zimbabwe[10]	7.6 (5/66)	1987
Kings County Medical Center[11]	13.6 (15/110)	1988
Grady Memorial Hospital[12]	15 (3/20)	1991
Mt. Sinai Medical Center[13]	16.7 (5/30)	1989
Kenyatta National Hospital[14]	20.9 (41/196)	1989
University Med. Center-Jacksonville[15]	22 (2/9)	1991

Diagnosis

The sensitivity and specificity of the clinical diagnosis of PID is woefully inadequate. The accuracy of the clinical and laboratory criteria used to diagnose PID may be further compromised by HIV infection associated with significant immunocompromise. For example, erythrocyte sedimentation rate, a laboratory parameter commonly elevated in women with PID, increases with advancing HIV disease. The World Health Organization (WHO) International Collaborating Group reported significantly lower erythrocyte sedimentation rate (ESR) in early stage HIV (95% confidence interval range from 11.4–16.3) than in stage 3 (27.0–38.1) or stage 4 disease (43.2–53.0).[16] Rompalo and coworkers reported lower sensitivity of cervical gram stain for diagnosis of *N. gonorrhoeae* infections among HIV+ women compared with HIV− (32% vs. 70%).[17] Decreasing peripheral blood counts are to be expected as the immune system is affected in the course of HIV progression. Therefore, these tests may be of even less value in the diagnostic criteria for PID among HIV-infected women.

Two reports in the literature address the issue of clinical presentation of PID in HIV-infected women. The first, compared 15 HIV+ women and 95 HIV− women with PID.[11] The two groups were similar in age and parity. Injection drug use was noted in 6 of the 15 HIV+ women. Admitting white blood cell counts (WBCs) greater than 10,000/mm^3 was reported in 40% of the HIV+ women compared with 89% of HIV− women. There was no significant difference between HIV+ and HIV− women in the number presenting with fever. A trend towards more syphilis infections was noted in the HIV seropositive group. *N. gonorrhoeae* and *C. trachomatis* infections were found in 33% and 15% of HIV+ compared with 25% and 16% of HIV− women. These differences were not statistically significant. In a second report, we published data on 23 HIV+ and 108 HIV− women with PID.[18] These groups of women were similar in age, gravidity, parity, race, drug use, multiple sexual partners, cigarette smoking, and history of prior episodes of PID. Injection drug use was reported by 78% of the HIV+ and 20% of the HIV− women ($p < 0.01$). On admission physical examination, the HIV+ women had significantly less abdominal tenderness but similar pelvic tenderness using a modified McCormack scale. Admission and discharge peripheral WBCs were lower in the HIV+ women with PID (HIV+: 8.97, 5.67, HIV−: 13.17, 7.41). There was also a trend toward higher ESRs in the HIV+ group (43.9 vs. 33.2).

Neisseria gonorrhoeae and *C. trachomatis* infections were found in 27% and 0% of HIV+ compared with 40% and 12% of HIV− patients. These were both statistically significant differences. This difference in peripheral WBCs may be explained in part, but not completely, by the lower frequency of *N. gonorrhoeae* infections in the HIV+ group.

Several additional studies have been presented at national and international conferences. Irwin and coworkers[19] compared 30 HIV+ and 127

HIV− women with PID-seeking treatment in emergency departments in New York City and Miami. The groups had similar pelvic tenderness scores but cervical friability, genital or anal ulcers, reactive syphilis tests, positive urine cultures, elevated C-reactive protein, adnexal masses on sonogram, and elevated ESRs were all more common in the HIV+ group. They noted that similar proportions of the HIV+ and HIV− women had taken analgesics before admission but that the HIV+ women were more likely to have taken antibiotics before admission. This could explain differences in microbiological tests between the HIV+ and HIV− groups. In another study, Munkolenkole and coworkers[20] reported findings in 57 HIV+ compared with 113 HIV− women with PID in Abidjan, Ivory Coast. The HIV+ women were more likely to have fever, vaginal discharge, genital ulcers, and tubo-ovarian abscesses.

Clinical Course and Treatment

A number of factors including alteration of vaginal flora, decreased mucosal immune function in the vagina, endocervix and endometrium or systemic immune suppression could all potentially influence the clinical course of PID in HIV-infected women. A twofold increase in the presence of vaginal anaerobes in HIV+ compared with HIV− prostitutes has been reported by Friedmann et al.[21] In another report, HIV was identified by in situ hybridization in the endometrium of a woman with refractory menometrorrhagia.[22] This patient had a lymphocytic and plasma cell infiltrate with no pathogenic organism noted on special stains. Johnstone et al.[23] reported on endometrial samples taken from 12 HIV+ and 11 HIV− women. The HIV+ group had increased CD45+ cells and CD3+ cells but decreased CD4+ cells compared to the HIV− group. These changes preceded the onset of clinically detectable immune suppression. This may indicate a decreased cellular immune response in the endometrium of HIV-infected women, which could lead to increased susceptibility to endometrial infection, increased colonization by pathogenic bacteria, or decreased clinical response once infection is established. The increased numbers of CD3+ cells may indicate a chronic endometrial infection. These authors speculate that this could account for the high rate (27% per year) of symptomatic PID in their cohort of 195 HIV+ women. Moorman and coworkers[24] compared endometrial biopsy histopathology and microbiology in 5 HIV+ and 46 HIV− women with PID. Endometritis was more frequent in HIV+ (67%) than in HIV− (12%) women. However, the low rate of endometritis in the HIV− women with PID is considerably lower than others have reported. Our report, described more endometrial *N. gonorrhoeae* and *C. trachomatis* infections in the HIV+ group despite equal frequency of cervical infections.[18] Endometrial anaerobic infection was less common in HIV+ (0/5) than HIV− (7/46). women. This group of studies suggest that there may be alterations in endometrial immunity in HIV+ women that could lead to differences in colonization with anaerobic bacteria and spread of a variety of microorganisms to the upper genital tract.

There is limited data describing the course of PID in HIV-infected women. Hoegsberg and coworkers[11] found a trend to more surgical intervention in HIV+ than in HIV− women (27% vs. 8% $p = 0.06$). The four HIV+ women who required surgical treatment in this study had persistent fevers refractory to antibiotic treatment. Two were treated with salpingo-oophorectomy, 1 with hysterectomy and salpingo-oophorectomy, and 1 with laparoscopic drainage. The length of antibiotic treatment and hospitalization was similar in the two groups. There was a trend toward more tubo-ovarian abscesses in the HIV+ compared with the HIV− group (23% vs. 14%, $p = 0.24$).

At San Francisco General Hospital, we found similar lengths of hospitalization and durations of antimicrobial treatment among HIV+ and HIV− patients.[18] Surgical intervention was required in 4 (17%) of the HIV+ compared with 4 (4%) of the HIV− patients ($p < 0.05$). This occurred despite the lower frequency of tubo-ovarian abscess in the HIV+ (4%) than in the HIV− (13%) patients. Surgical therapy consisted of hysterectomy and salpingo-oophorectomy in all cases and was performed for failed resolution of fever or symptomatic improvement despite antibiotic therapy. Three of the 4 HIV+ patients requiring surgery had AIDS. Women with asymptomatic HIV infection required surgical treatment no more frequently than HIV− women although the study's statistical power was insufficient to validate this finding.

To date, three additional studies have been presented in abstract form. Barbosa and coworkers[25] compared 12 HIV+ and 139 HIV− patients admitted to Kings County Hospital in Brooklyn, New York between 7/92 and 3/92. The HIV+ women had lower peripheral WBCs and required longer hospitalization than the HIV− women. One of the 12 HIV+ women, the only one with AIDS in this group, required surgical treatment. There was no difference between groups stratified for positive urine toxicology. Irwin and coworkers[19] found HIV+ women were as likely to be admitted for treatment of PID as HIV− women but once admitted had rates of clinical improvement similar to HIV− women. Surgical treatment was required in 10% of the HIV+ and 4% of the HIV− groups. This difference was not statistically significant. Munkolenkole et al. reported findings in 57 HIV+ compared with 113 HIV− women with PID in Abidjan, Ivory Coast. Surgical intervention was necessary in HIV+ women more frequently than HIV− women (OR 6.5, 95% CI 1.1, 67.5).[20] In those who did not require surgery, the clinical course was similar to that of HIV− women.

In summary, the studies described here suggest that the clinical presentation and course of PID in HIV+ women may differ from that in HIV− women. This appears to be most significant and perhaps only significant among women with symptomatic HIV disease and/or severe immune suppression.

Well-controlled studies with stratification of patients by measures of immune function such as CD4+ counts are needed to determine if any of the differences suggested by the current studies are valid. The current data support the Centers for Disease Control recommendation that HIV+ women with PID receive inpatient treatment with standard antibiotic regimens.[26] Whether other measures will improve outcome in AIDS patients with PID is unknown at present.

References

1. 1993 Revised Classification System for HIV infection and expanded surveillance case definition for AIDS among adolescents and adults. *JAMA* 1993; **269**:729–730.

2. Laga M, Monoka A, Kivuvu M, et al. Non-ulcerative sexually transmitted diseases as risk factors for HIV-1 transmission in women: Results from a cohort study. *AIDS* 1993;**7**(1):95–102.

3. Saracco A, Musicco M, Nicolosi A, et al. Man to woman transmission of HIV: Longitudinal study of 343 steady partners of infected men. *JAIDS* 1993;**6**:497–502.

4 Plummer FA, Simonsen JN, Cameron DW, Ndinya-Achola JO, Kreiss JK, Gakinya MN, Waiyaki P, Cheang M, Piot P, Ronald AR, et al. Cofactors in male-female sexual transmission of human immunodeficiency virus type 1. *J Inf Dis* 1991;**163**(2):233–239.

5. Cohen CR, Pruithithada N, Rugpao S, et al. Relationship between bacterial vaginosis and HIV seropositivity among female commercial sex workers in Chiang Mai, Thailand, in *First National Conference on Human Retroviruses and Related Infections*. Washington, DC, December, 1993. Abstract 155.

6. Futterman D, Cohn J, Moraru R, Monte D, Hein K. HIV+ adolescents: STD's and gynecologic findings in a New York City cohort, in *IX International Conference on AIDS*. Berlin, June, 1993. Abstract PO-B11-1526.

7. Clark RA, Brandon W, Dumestre J, Pindaro C. Clinical manifestations of infection with the human immunodeficiency virus in women in Louisiana. *Clin Inf Dis* 1993;**17**:165–172.

8. Friedland IR, Klugman KP, Karstaedt AS, Patel J, McIntyre JA, Allwood CW. AIDS—the Baragwanath experience. *S Afr Med J* 1992;**82**:86–90.

9. Safrin S, Dattel BJ, Hauer L, Sweet RL. Seroprevalence and epidemiologic correlates of human immunodeficiency virus infection in women with acute pelvic inflammatory disease. *Obstet Gynecol* 1990;**75**:666–670.

10. Muylder ZD, Laga M, Tennstedt C, Van Dyck E, Aelbers GNM, Piot P. The role of *Neisseria gonorrhoeae* and *Chlamydia trachomatis* in pelvic inflammatory disease and its sequelae in Zimbabwe. *J Infect Dis* 1990;**162**:501–505.

11. Hoegsberg B, Abulafia O, Sedlis A, et al. Sexually transmitted diseases and human immunodeficiency virus among women with pelvic inflammatory disease. *Am J Obstet Gynecol* 1990;**163**:1135–1139.

12. Lindsay MK, Grant J, Peterson HB, Risby J, Williams H, Klein L. Human immunodeficiency virus infection among patients in a gynecology emergency room. *Obstet Gynecol* 1993;**81**:1012–1015.

13. Sperling RS, Friedman F, Joyner M, Brodman M, Dottino P. Seroprevalence of human immunodeficiency virus in women admitted to the hospital with pelvic inflammatory disease. *J Reprod Med* 1991;**36**:122–124.

14 Ojwang AW, Lema VW, Wanjala SHM. HIV infection among patients with acute pelvic inflammatory disease at the Kenyatta national hospital, Nairobi, Kenya. *E Afr Med J* 1993;**70**:506–511.

15. Shannon J, Benrubi GI. Epidemiology of pelvic inflammatory disease at University Medical Center, Jacksonville. *J Fla Med Assoc* 1991;**78**:158–161.

16. The WHO International Collaborating Group. Proposed World Health Organization staging system for HIV infection and disease: preliminary testing by an international collaborative cross-sectional study. *AIDS* 1993;**7**:711–718.

17. Rompalo A, Lawler J, Williamson B, Brown R, Woltmann M, Zenilman J. Impact of HIV on clinical manifestations of STDs among women attending Baltimore STD clinics, in *33rd Interscience Conference on Antimicrobial Agents and Chemotherapy*. New Orleans, LA, 1993. Abstract 1167.

18. Korn AP, Landers DV, Green JR, Sweet RL. Pelvic inflammatory disease in human immunodeficiency virus-infected women. *Obstet Gynecol* 1993;**82**: 765–768.

19. Irwin K, Rice R, O'Sullivan M, Sperling R, Brodman M, Moorman A. The influence of HIV infection on initial symptoms and course of pelvic inflammatory disease: Updated results of an ongoing multicenter study, in *Infectious Disease Society for Obstetrics and Gynecology, Annual Meeting*. Monterey, CA, August, 1994.

20. Munkolenkole K, De Cock KM, St Louis M, Ghys P, Touré CK, Kreiss J. HIV infection is associated with more severe clinical presentation of PID, in *Xth International Conference on AIDS*. Yokohama, Japan, August, 1994. Abstract PB0788.

21. Friedmann W, Schafer APS, Schwartlander B. Opportunistic diseases in HIV infected women, in *IX International Conference on AIDS*. Berlin, June, 1993. Abstract WS-B17-3.

22. Peuchmaur M, Emilie D, Vazeux R, et al. HIV-associated endometrtis. *AIDS* 1989;**3**:239–241.

23. Johnstone FD, Williams ARW, Bird GA, Bjornsson S. Immunohistochemical characterization of endometrial lymphoid cell populations in women infected with human immunodeficiency virus. *Obstet Gynecol* 1994;**83**:586–593.

24. Moorman A, Rice R, Irwin K, O'Sullivan M, Sperling R, Brodman M and the Multicenter HIV and PID study group. The microbiologic etiology of pelvic inflammatory disease in HIV+ and HIV− women: Updated results from an ongoing multi-center study, in *First National Conference on Human Retroviruses and Related Infections*. Washington, DC, December, 1993. Abstract 252.

25. Barbosa C, Duerr A, Brockmann S, Macasaet M, Clarke L, Minkhoff H. Clinical course of pelvic inflammatory disease in HIV infected women. Infectious Disease Society for Obstetrics and Gynecology. Stowe, VT, August, 1993.

26. Centers for Disease Control. 1993 Sexually transmitted diseases treatment guidelines. *MMWR* 1993;**42**:RR-14.

10
Prevention of Pelvic Inflammatory Disease

Julius Schachter

Prevention of pelvic inflammatory disease (PID) has two major goals. The first is to prevent the morbidity, time lost from work, pain, suffering, and medical costs associated with acute PID. The second goal is to prevent the long-term consequences of PID. Late sequelae of this condition are important medically and to society. Approximately 20% of women are rendered infertile after an episode of PID and the risks of ectopic pregnancy are increased 6- to 10-fold.[1] Chronic pelvic pain is another long-term consequence.

Because approximately 65% to 75% of acute episodes of PID can be associated with common sexually transmitted bacterial pathogens, *Chlamydia trachomatis* and *Neisseria gonorrhoeae*, it is obvious that prevention of sexually transmitted diseases (STDs) is a major component in prevention of PID.[2] Indeed, most of the risk factors for PID are the same as those identified for STDs. However, serological studies of the relationship of *C. trachomatis* to tubal factor infertility and ectopic pregnancy have shown that most of the women who suffer these late consequences of PID have high titers of antichlamydial antibody as compared to appropriate controls (pregnant women or women who are infertile for other reasons), but that the majority have no antecedent history of PID.[3,4]

A number of clinical studies have found chlamydial PID to be clinically milder than gonococcal PID or nonchlamydial, nongonococcal PID.[5] The seroepidemiological findings on late consequences of PID, together with detection of ascending infection in asymptomatic women exposed to chlamydia and persistent upper genital tract infection in women inadequately treated after a clinical episode of PID, have all contributed to the concept of inapparent salpingitis caused by *C. trachomatis*.[6,7] Given that a clinically inapparent tubal infection can be associated with the long-term consequences of PID, it is even more important that STDs be prevented generically. In other words, to prevent PID one must prevent the STDs. The approaches to STD prevention include attempts to reduce the reservoir and thus reduce exposures, as well as specific intervention modalities that can be aimed at individuals. Basically, these stress education and communication.

Some of the risk factors associated with STDs and PID are not amenable to intervention or prevention. For example, race and socioeconomic status can be associated with both. The frequency of intercourse in monogamous relationships is associated with PID,[8] but it is unreasonable to assume that we can inform women that they should be having sex less often, as a PID preventative. There are, however, a number of points that can be communicated to women that would prevent PID or reduce attack rates for PID; that many of them are the same messages we would like to communicate for reduction of STDs is, in fact, beneficial. It emphasizes the legitimacy of the STD prevention message when the target population is informed that they are doing something to protect themselves (or to preserve their fertility) rather than getting a message that they should be doing something to prevent urethritis in men.

Some of the messages are simple, but the fact that they are simple does not mean that they are easily implemented. For example, delaying the onset of sexual activity is desirable to reduce STD rates and prevent PID. Younger women are at higher risk for STDs, and in a population, young women are at greatest risk for development of acute salpingitis.[1,2] Similarly, for those who are sexually active, placing the emphasis on monogamy, rather than having multiple partners is important in reducing STDs and PID, as multiple partners and acquisition of new partners are risk factors for acquisition of STDs and development of PID.[9]

A major thrust in STD prevention programs is the promotion of condom usage. The use of barrier contraceptive methods (condoms, diaphragms, and spermicidal jellies) is associated with a reduction in the risk of development of PID.[2]

The above points focus on the reduction in acquisition of STDs, particularly *N. gonorrhoeae* and *C. trachomatis*. That certainly should be the major focus because it is obvious that we do not know when an infection reaches the oviducts. Clearly women with classical presentations of acute salpingitis have such a disease. While we do not understand the pathogenesis of PID, it seems reasonable to suggest that early intensive chemotherapy when lower genital tract infections are identified is desirable. Even if some proportion of women with apparently uncomplicated lower genital tract infections may already have silent upper genital tract infections, some may not yet have such infections and would benefit by early therapy to prevent ascendancy. Thus, it is important for women who have multiple partners to know they are at risk for asymptomatic infection and that they should be screened for such infections on a regular basis, perhaps at the time of annual gynecological examinations. Parallel with this thought, it is incumbent upon clinicians dealing with patients who may be at risk for STDs to be aware of that risk, to know how to ask the relevant questions, and to perform appropriate diagnostic tests. Similarly, patient and clinician should be aware of the symptoms of lower genital tract disease. Women should be educated as to the nature of abnormal symptoms that require medical care. This knowledgeable clientele requires that we have well-educated clinicians. Appropriate health-care-seeking behavior by women in response to symptoms such as vaginal discharge and lower abdominal pain, dyspareunia, etc. demands an appropriate response by the clinicians.

Each partner should assume the responsibility of informing the other if symptoms appear or an STD is diagnosed. A woman who has such symptoms should immediately cease sexual activity to prevent transmission of infections to partner(s). The male partner should understand that if he develops signs or symptoms of genital tract disease he should immediately notify his partner. If either partner is diagnosed with an STD, sexual activity should stop and diagnostic tests and appropriate treatment for partners should be initiated. Contact tracing should be a high priority for health providers and public health agencies. It is imperative that all infected individuals receive appropriate therapy, and that they understand how long they should be taking the pills, how many pills should be taken, what the requirements are for test-of-cure, when they can initiate sexual activity, and under what circumstances.

These are the features that are clearly associated with STD control and that relate to prevention of PID. There are some other issues that are not clear at all. The role of oral contraceptives (OCs) in preventing PID is not clear.[10] There are many studies showing higher cervical chlamydial infection rates in women on OCs. There are also studies showing that women on OCs have milder upper genital tract disease when they develop PID, or that there may be protective effects preventing development of PID.[9] If, however, chlamydial salpingitis tends to be milder under any circumstances, and OCs tend to further reduce symptoms, it is possible that OCs increase the tendency toward more asymptomatic PID.

There are a number of features of PID that are amenable to specific preventive efforts. For example, it is known that intrauterine device (IUD) usage is associated with higher rates of PID.[11] An intervention may be specific for the demographic attributes of the patient. For example, an IUD may be perfectly acceptable for a 40-year-old multiparous woman who has no interest in having more children and who smokes and has phlebitis. However, the IUD would be inappropriate for use by a nulliparous teenager who might have multiple or even serial partners. It is also clear that there is a relatively high risk of developing PID within 3 or 4 months of insertion of the IUD. This is usually attributed to introduction of vaginal flora into the sterile uterine cavity, thus allowing the organisms access to the fallopian tube. It is possible that prophylactic antibiotics may be useful in this context, that is, given at time of insertion of the IUD. Certainly prophylaxis is called for in selected subsets of women having abortions. Postabortal PID rates have been dramatically reduced by screening women prior to the abortion and treating those found to be infected with chlamydia with a tetracycline to prevent subsequent development of PID.[12] But not all women having elective abortion are routinely tested for chlamydia. The recommendation for routine screening of women for chlamydial infection prior to abortion may be appropriate in some populations. It may also be useful to test for bacterial vaginosis (BV) in this setting.[13]

Bacterial vaginosis may also be considered a risk factor for development of PID.[14] It is certainly not proven, but it is an attractive hypothesis to consider that many of the upper genital tract infections with non-STD pathogens represent the perturbed flora seen in BV. Perhaps BV in the presence of a permeable endocervical canal (caused either by timing in the menstrual cycle, or by damage due to chlamydial or gonococcal infection, or IUD string) allows ascendance of flora to the upper genital tract. Some data suggest that intercourse during menses is a risk factor for ascending infection. Thus, avoiding such timing of coitus may be a reasonable recommendation.

Vaginal douching is another behavior that can be associated with increased risk of PID.[15] Douching has also been associated with tubal damage (ectopic pregnancy) in women without history of PID.[16] This suggests that asymptomatic or inapparent PID can be caused by organisms other than *C. trachomatis*. Given that there are relatively few medical indications for douching it seems reasonable to recommend that douching not be done except under specific orders from a clinician, particularly in women with other risk factors for PID.

The ultimate goal of PID prevention is really to minimize the consequences of PID—ectopic pregnancy and tubal factor infertility. While not directly related to preventing PID, one would be remiss in not mentioning that early and effective antimicrobial treatment of symptomatic PID has been shown to prevent these consequences.[17] Thus, it would be important to inform women about the early signs and symptoms of PID and the importance of seeking medical attention soon after the symptoms begin.

There are data to suggest that smoking is a risk factor for development of PID and its consequences.[2] Obviously, smoking cessation is a desirable goal from many viewpoints and is unlikely to be part of PID control programs.

Certainly biological preventive measures could play an important role, but it is unlikely that effective vaccines for chlamydial or gonococcal infections will be available in the near future. Thus, as noted above, although there are some preventive measures specific for PID, a broad-based program will be based on a general STD prevention program. There will be a greater stress on screening of asymptomatic populations. While we have the biological tools to use in such a program, it is unrealistic to expect a successful PID control program until our society is willing to take responsibility for one. This means more than a simple financial commitment, although a control program will be expensive. What is required is a commitment to a philosophy of prevention, as opposed to crisis management. The commitment here must be for a cohesive and collaborative program integrating the different facets of our health community that can contribute to the preventive approach. Certainly the home is where such efforts should be initiated, and educational materials should be made available to parents. However, it is ludicrous to depend exclusively upon the family setting when one of our major concerns is lack of education for physicians and other health-care providers. Thus STD (and PID) prevention must be the shared concern of multiple facets of our society. Starting with the family, then through the schools and the media, and from the physician, other health-care workers, and public health agencies must come the messages. Education will be a crucial preventive measure, and ultimately it is the shared responsibility of each of these groups. All must play a role in prevention.

References

1. Weström L. Incidence, prevalence and trends of acute pelvic inflammatory disease and its consequences in industrialized countries. *Am J Obstet Gynecol* 1980;**138**:880.
2. Washington AE, Aral SO, Wølner-Hanssen P, Grimes DA, Holmes KK. Assessing risk for pelvic inflammatory disease and its sequelae. *JAMA* **266**(18):2581–2586.
3. Cates W Jr. Sexually transmitted organisms and infertility: The proof of the pudding. *Sex Transm Dis* 1984;**11**(2):113–116.
4. Cates W Jr, Wasserheit JN. Genital chlamydial infections: Epidemiology and reproductive sequelae. *Am J Obstet Gynecol* 1991;**164**:1771–1781.
5. Weström L, Mardh P-A. Acute pelvic inflammatory disease (PID), in Holmes KK, Mardh P-A, Sparling PF, Wiesner PJ (eds): *Sexually Transmitted Diseases*, 2nd ed. New York, McGraw-Hill Information Services Co., 1990, pp 593–613.
6. Sweet RL, Schachter J, Robbie M. Failure of beta lactam antibiotics to eradicate *Chlamydia trachomatis* in the endometrium despite apparent clinical cure of acute salpingitis. *JAMA* 1983;**250**(19):2641–2645.
7. Jones RB, Mammel JB, Shepard MK, Fisher RR. Recovery of *Chlamydia trachomatis* from the endometrium of women at risk for chlamydial infection. *Am J Obstet Gynecol* 1986;**155**(1):35.
8. Lee NC, Rubin GL, Grimes DA. Measures of sexual behavior and the risk of pelvic inflammatory disease. *Obstet Gynecol* 1991;**77**(3):425–430.
9. Wølner-Hanssen P, Eschenbach DA, Paavonen J, Kiviat N, Stevens CE, Critchlow C, DeRouen T, Holmes KK. Decreased risk of symptomatic chlamydial pelvic inflammatory disease associated with oral contraceptives use. *JAMA* 1990;**263**(1):54–59.
10. Washington AE, Gove S, Schachter J, Sweet RL. Oral contraceptives and *Chlamydia* infections. Letters. *JAMA* 1986;**255**(1):38–39.
11. World Health Organization. *Mechanism of Action, Safety and Efficacy of Intrauterine Devices.* Geneva, Switzerland: World Health Organization; 1987. Technical report series 753.
12. Osser S, Persson K. Postabortal infectious morbidity after antibiotic treatment of chlamydia-positive patients. *Sex Transm Dis* 1989;**16**(2):84–87.
13. Spiegel CA. Bacterial vaginosis. *Clin Microb Reviews* 1991;**4**(4):485–502.

14. Larsson P-G, Platz-Christensen J-J, Thejls H, Forsum U, Pahlson C. Incidence of pelvic inflammatory disease after first-trimester legal abortion in women with bacterial vaginosis after treatment with metronidazole: A double-blind, randomized study. *Am J Obstet Gynecol* 1992;**166**(1):100–103.

15. Wølner-Hanssen P, Eschenbach DA, Paavonen J, et al. Association between vaginal douching and acute pelvic inflammatory disease. *JAMA* 1990;**263**: 1936–1941.

16. Chow JM, Yonekura L, Richwald GA, Greenland S, Sweet RL, Schachter J. The association between *Chlamydia trachomatis* and ectopic pregnancy: A matched-pair, case-control study. *JAMA* 1990;**263**:3164–3167.

17. Hillis SD, Joesoef R, Marchbanks PA, Wasserheit JN, Cates W Jr., Weström L. Delayed care of pelvic inflammatory disease as a risk factor for impaired fertility. *Am J Obstet Gynecol* 1993;**168**(5):1503–1509.

11
Long-term Sequelae of Pelvic Inflammatory Disease: Tubal Factor Infertility, Ectopic Pregnancy, and Chronic Pelvic Pain

JOAN M. CHOW AND JULIUS SCHACHTER

In pelvic inflammatory disease (PID) there is a process of tissue destruction and scarring that, in the absence of aggressive treatment, may lead to irrevocable changes in fallopian tubal morphology. The implications for subsequent fertility have been recognized since the last century. Women with untreated or inadequately treated pelvic infections due to sexually transmitted diseases (STDs) are less fertile.[1] With the use of follow-up studies, three major sequelae of symptomatic PID have been identified: tubal factor infertility (TFI), ectopic pregnancy, and chronic pelvic pain.[2-4] Results from seroepidemiological studies have associated similar sequelae with "silent" or unrecognized PID.[5] Animal models of PID pathogenesis have also provided some additional data on the development of sequelae. The considerable physical and economic cost ($1 billion in the United States in 1990) associated with these sequelae further justifies greater efforts to develop intervention strategies to prevent PID.[6]

Tubal Factor Infertility

Infertility is commonly defined as the failure to conceive after 1 year of unprotected intercourse.[7] Tubal factor infertility is due to a functional impairment of the fallopian tube involving adhesions, scarring and occlusion, which may be confirmed by macroscopic examination, hysterosalpingography, or laparoscopy. Observations by physicians earlier in this century documented the diminished fertility that often followed an acute episode of salpingitis. The reported fertility rate after salpingitis in married couples ranged from 25% to 80%.[8-12] Although these reports did not rule out other physical causes of involuntary fertility (e.g., male factor infertility) post-PID infertility was well recognized.

Concurrent PID and TFI

Several investigators have tried to demonstrate a possible concurrent relationship between PID and TFI; that is, could active or persistent infection

152

with PID organisms result in tubal damage leading to infertility? A series of studies by Henry-Suchet and colleagues[13–16] reported the isolation of *Chlamydia trachomatis* (15% to 35%) as well as various other aerobic-anaerobic bacteria (Mycoplasmas, *Bacteroides* species) from the tubes, adhesions, or peritoneum of women with TFI and no clinical signs of PID. Laparoscopy was used to identify a chronic inflammatory condition described by the authors as "a yellowish viscous, abundant effusion of Douglas' cul de sac, and the viscous, red, and brilliant appearance of the peritoneum surfaces and of the adhesions," also described as "a viscous pelvis." From this group of TFI patients, 23.3% were culture-positive for *C. trachomatis*, versus 15.4% of TFI patients without this inflammatory condition and 2% of infertile controls with normal tubes. TFI patients with tubal inflammation were also more likely to be seropositive (1:20–1:160 IgG) for *C. trachomatis* (57.1%) than controls (20%).

While the French studies strongly suggested that a concurrent or chronic clinically inapparent tubal infection due to *C. trachomatis* and/or other organisms may be responsible for the failure to conceive, other studies of tubal or cervical cultures from TFI patients have not duplicated the results. In one study by Shepherd and Jones,[17] only the use of multiple passages enabled the isolation of chlamydial organisms from endometrial and tube biopsies in 8 of 52 TFI patients. With the advent of nonculture diagnostic tests for *C. trachomatis* in particular, there has been further exploration of the persistent PID issue among TFI patients. Thejls and colleagues[18] used a direct fluorescent antibody (DFA) test and two enzyme immunoassays (EIA) for antigen detection, as well as cultures and serology to study infertile women undergoing tuboplasty or laparoscopy. Eight percent of 256 TFI patients had ten or more chlamydial elementary bodies (EBs) per smears from the cervix, endometrium, and fallopian tubes; six patients had either a positive chlamydial culture or direct antigen test (all six had high EB counts). Campbell and colleagues[19] used in situ hybridization and immunoperoxidase (IP) staining to detect *C. trachomatis* in the fallopian tube tissues of infertile women with distal tubal occlusion. *C. trachomatis* DNA or antigen was detected in 9 of 16 culture-negative infertile cases, which led to the suggestion that the organism can persist in the tube in an uncultivable state. In contrast, tubal biopsies from 6 control patients with normal fallopian tubes, no prior PID history, and sero-negative for chlamydial antibodies were all negative by these two methods. It remains to be seen if the use of polymerase chain reaction and ligase chain reaction technology[20] may increase our ability to detect the presence of PID organisms in specimens from the upper genital tract of TFI patients.

Part of the variability in microbiological results is likely due to how the infertility cases are identified. In the French cases, it is likely that these women are referred directly to an infertility specialist after a period of unprotected intercourse. It is likely that many of these women have silent or unrecognized salpingitis. In contrast, in the United States, infertility cases are the subjects of study at tertiary health-care settings, and have likely been diagnosed and treated by their gynecologists, after which they are referred for further evaluations. These women are more likely to have old "burnt out" disease. Reports of relevant pathological findings would help to define the status of the patients' disease.

Follow-up Studies

A series of follow-up studies of women with a laparoscopically verified diagnosis of PID to determine subsequent fertility experience was performed over a span of more than 20 years by Weström and colleagues in Lund, Sweden.[21-23] These logistically difficult studies provide the most convincing estimates of risk associated with PID sequelae because they were done with a homogeneous, stable population with consistent medical follow-up over a long period of time. Approximately 1700 cases of PID and 600 control patients were followed after a diagnostic laparoscopy during the period from 1960 to 1984. Tubal factor infertility was defined as infertility caused by tubal occlusion verified by hysterosalpingography, laparoscopy, laparotomy, or a combination of the above. Of those who exposed themselves to a chance of pregnancy, 16.0% of cases and 0% of the controls had confirmed TFI. The rate of TFI was directly associated with severity and number of PID episodes. Each repeated episode of PID roughly doubled the TFI rate. These findings were not affected by the change in PID treatment regimens over the 20 years because there was a constant proportion of women with TFI associated with PID each year.

Prospective studies on the scale of the Swedish studies are difficult and expensive to conduct in the absence of a highly centralized medical care system with stable populations and extensive follow-up. There have been two studies since then that have attempted to measure the risk of infertility following PID. One concurrent follow-up study of PID patients was conducted by Adler and colleagues.[24] After 21 months of follow-up, PID patients did not experience more infertility than control patients, a finding not consistent with the Swedish studies, and perhaps due to the short follow-up.

Longer follow-up was obtained by Safrin and colleagues[25] who conducted a retrospective cohort study in which 140 patients identified by chart review as having a discharge diagnosis of PID were contacted after a median time of 37 months. Forty one percent of patients were involuntarily infertile, and history of PID before admission was a significant risk factor.

Retrospective Studies

Chlamydial Infections and TFI

There have been numerous retrospective studies reported in which seroepidemiological methods were used. These studies identified women with and without tubal factor infertility and measured the proportion of those with IgG antibodies to *C. trachomatis*. The proportion of women with TFI and antichlamydial antibodies ranged from 57% to 86% versus only 0% to 25% of women who are infertile for other reasons or who have no tubal disease.[26-34] The relative risk of TFI associated with past exposure to *C. trachomatis* ($\geq 1:64$ IgG) has been estimated to be as high as 7.8 (95% Cl: 3.2–19.1) after adjustment for age,[35] although it has been 3–4 in most studies. The level of chlamydial antibodies has also been directly related to the severity of tubal damage and pelvic adhesions seen on diagnostic laparoscopy.

Further serological studies have been done using assays to detect antibody response to the chlamydial heat shock protein (Chsp60) in TFI patients. Chlamydial heat shock protein is thought to induce a delayed hypersensitivity response in animal models and it has been assumed that it is important in tissue damage caused by *C. trachomatis*.[36] Toye and colleagues[37] found that 84% of TFI patients had Chsp60 antibodies versus 20% of prenatal patients.

It is important to note that in most of these serological studies, only 10% to 15% of the women with antichlamydial antibodies reported either any past clinical symptoms suggestive of PID or a confirmed diagnosis of PID. It is particularly through the use of retrospective seroepidemiological studies that we have arrived at the concept of silent or "atypical" PID associated with chlamydial infection leading to TFI sequelae. Any prevention measures aimed at reducing the incidence of PID and associated sequelae will also need to identify factors associated with asymptomatic as well as clinical PID. In a study by Mueller and colleagues,[38] 33 infertile women with no previous history of PID were compared with 129 infertile women with such a history and 501 fertile women. Factors such as use of the Dalkon Shield™ intrauterine device (IUD) and other types of IUD were associated with silent PID in tubal infertile women. In contrast, use of oral contraceptives (OCs) for longer than 3 years was associated with a decreased risk of silent disease. Confirmation of exposure to PID organisms by cultures or serology was not done.

Role of Other Organisms and TFI

While there is substantial evidence to implicate past chlamydial infection as a risk factor for TFI,[39] few studies have looked at past exposure to gonococcal and mycoplasmal infections in the same analysis with data on chlamydial exposure to determine whether they may be independently or sequentially related to TFI. This is partly due to the lack of specific and sensitive serological tests. Studies from western Europe and central Africa[40-46] have all found high prevalences of antibodies to these three organisms among TFI cases. The prevalence of antibody to *Neisseria gonorrhoeae* and *Mycoplasma hominis* was shown to be as high as 61% and 75%, respectively, among cases from the Netherlands.[41] Among TFI cases from the Gambia, 89% of cases had antibodies to either gonococcal antigens or chlamydial antigens or both, as compared with 46% of matched pregnant controls.[40] Møller and colleagues reported that *M. hominis* antibodies were found significantly more frequently in infertile women with abnormal hysterosalpingography results.[46] In addition, Miettinen[45] found that 72% of TFI cases with abnormal tubes were seropositive to one or more of the these organisms as compared with 21% of infertile controls with normal tubes. The serological findings confirmed that women with gonococcal PID are more likely to clinical episodes: half of the women who were seropositive for gonococcal infection in Miettinen's study reported past PID symptoms versus 25% of the women with positive chlamydial or mycoplasmal serology. In the case of *M. hominis* exposure, the association with TFI was limited to those women with secondary infertility. This exposure to *M. hominis* may have occurred during complications of pregnancy and delivery.

Substantial interest has been generated in the association of anaerobes with PID. Anaerobes have been isolated from the upper genital tract in PID patients. However, it has been unclear whether their presence reflects a pathogenic role or perturbed vaginal flora in bacterial vaginosis (BV). In PID cases where gonococci and chlamydia are not identified, anaerobes may be important. However, there are no large-scale studies of anaerobes in PID due to the difficulty of culture and lack of convenient, sensitive assays. Consequently, no studies have reported the risk of long-term sequelae associated with PID caused by anaerobes. This is an area that deserves further investigation.

Ectopic Pregnancy

Ectopic pregnancy (EP) is defined as the implantation of the blastocyst outside of the endometrial cavity in the following sites: fallopian tube, ovary, cervix, cornua, peritoneal cavity. The increased incidence of ectopic pregnancy in developed countries over the past 20 years has been a major focus of study.[47–52] The U.S. Centers for Disease Control (CDC), which began surveillance of ectopic pregnancy rates in 1970 has documented a fourfold rise in the EP rates over the past 20 years, from 4.5 to 16.0 ectopic pregnancies per 1,000 reported pregnancies.[53] The absolute number of cases per year has also risen fivefold, from 17,800 to 88,400.[53] While some of the increase may be due to the shift in age distribution for women in their childbearing years, use of the IUD and tubal ligation contraceptive methods, investigators have considered coincident rises in STD and PID rates to be major factors.[48,49,52] The post-PID functional impairment in the tube resulting from occlusion, scarring and adhesion is consistently found to be the strongest predictor of increased risk of tubal ectopic pregnancy.[21,39,48] In addition, it appears that recurrent infections with PID organisms such as *C. trachomatis* may also significantly increase the risk of TEP.[54]

Follow-up Studies

The PID follow-up studies from Lund, Sweden were also able to determine the incidence of ectopic pregnancy during the 25-year period after laparoscopically verified PID.[21,22] The results confirmed the strong relationship between PID and EP. The relative risk of EP was 7.0 after one PID episode, 16.6 after two episodes, and 28.3 after three or more PID episodes. Moreover, severity of PID also was directly related to EP risk: the relative risk of EP was 4.2 for mild PID, and 10.9 for severe PID.

Buchan and colleagues[55] reported the results of a follow-up study involving 1,355 hospitalized cases of PID from 1970–1985 compared with 10,507 hospital controls with other diagnoses. These patients' outcomes over the study period were tracked by means of computerized record linkage. This study, which provides a direct comparison with the Swedish studies, found similar results; PID cases were ten times as likely to be admitted for ectopic pregnancy.

The retrospective cohort study conducted by Safrin and colleagues[25] found that 2 EP (2.4%) cases were reported at 17 and 30 months post-PID admission, among the 51 patients. This constitutes an eightfold increase over the rate of EP observed in women of reproductive age in the general U.S. population.

Hillis and colleagues (54) also used a retrospective cohort design to determine the risk of EP associated with recurrent chlamydial infections. By linking a state disease surveillance registry with a hospital discharge database for the period 1985 to 1992, the authors were able to identify patients with episodes of chlamydial infection and subsequent treatment for EP. Compared to those with one chlamydial infection, women with 2 infections had a 2.5 -fold increased risk, and those with 3 or more infections had a five-fold increased risk of EP (estimates adjusted for demographic confounding factors). The gradient of effect is in the same direction as the Swedish studies, and suggests that the tissue damage leading to TEP is related to the chronic inflammation and scarring caused by repeated infection, rather than the primary infection.

Retrospective Studies

Chlamydial Infections and EP

Given the logistic difficulty of conducting comprehensive long-term follow-up studies of PID to measure EP incidence, investigators have been more successful at studying EP retrospectively using seroepidemiological methods. In most of these case-control studies, EP cases were compared to controls on the basis of IgG antibodies to *C. trachomatis*. Almost all studies reported that EP cases were significantly more likely to have antichlamydial antibodies than pregnant controls and previous exposure to *C. trachomatis* was associated with anywhere from a two- to fourfold increase in EP risk.[56-65] This risk estimate was unchanged in those studies that were able to control for confounding variables, such as age, race, parity, smoking, and douching. Three studies have studied whether chlamydial serological status is correlated with tubal histopathology among EP cases. Walters and colleagues[58] directly correlated serological titers with histologic and pathological changes in the affected tube. Brunham and colleagues[62] also found a direct relationship between plasma cell infiltration in the fallopian tubes and *C. trachomatis* seropositivity when comparing EP cases with tubal ligation controls (OR 7.2; 95%Cl, 1.7-31). Sheffield and colleagues[64] found that pelvic damage was associated with chlamydial serology with an adjusted odds ratio of 4.2 (95% Cl: 1.8-9.7) among EP cases. Moderate and severe pelvic damage was more strongly associated with positive serology than mild damage.

Further serological evidence of past exposure to specific chlamydial antigens such as (Chsp60) and *omp2* among PID and EP cases was reported by Wagar and colleagues.[66] In this study, while all the cases with high IgG titers ($\geq 1:512$) had antibody to *omp2*, 31.6% of the PID cases versus 81.0% of the EP cases had antibody to Chsp60. Brunham and colleagues[62] in the study of EP cases discussed above, also showed that the seropositive EP cases were more likely to have antibodies to chlamydial heat shock protein than seropositive tubal ligation controls. These studies suggest that women with PID with antibody to Chsp60 may be at higher risk of developing long-term chronic sequelae such as EP or TFI. However, the mechanism of this response is not well understood. Cell-mediated immune response to this antigen, in particular, is associated with the tubal damage leading to *C. trachomatis*-related ectopic pregnancy. However, immune response to Chsp60 may be only an indicator/marker of a chronic inflammatory process, and further study is warranted.

Other PID Organisms and EP

Seroepidemiological studies of EP have also considered the contribution of past exposure to *N. gonorrhoeae* and the mycoplasmas (*M. hominis* and *Ureaplasma urealyticum*) to a more limited extent than has been the case with *C. trachomatis*. As in the case with TFI, it is important to resolve the relative roles of these organisms as coinfections or subsequent infections with respect to the development to EP. Various studies from Europe and Africa have demonstrated a similar positive relationship between these infections and EP.[44,45,67] Robertson and colleagues reported that prevalence of gonococcal IgG antibody was 32% among EP cases versus 4%, which corresponds to a crude relative risk of 11.3 (95% Cl: 3.0-41.9).[67] However, in a study from Gabon, there was no statistical difference in gonococcal antibody levels between EP cases and pregnant controls.[68]

The role of the mycoplasmas in EP has received less attention. The rate of isolation of the mycoplasmas from the fallopian tubes and cul-de-sac fluid in PID cases has been relatively low[69] and it has not been possible to distinguish a pathogenic role in all cases. In contrast to *C. trachomatis* and *N. gonorrhoeae*, the mycoplasmas are normal flora of sexually active women, and may be found to be pathogenic on an opportunistic basis. In a case-control study by the authors and Dr. Gail Cassell, no relationship was found between *M. hominis* antibodies and ectopic pregnancy when exposure to *C. trachomatis* was taken into account (unpublished data). Other results by Miettinen[45] indicated that previous mycoplasmal PID exposure may be a factor in EP: 37% of infertile women with a history of ectopic pregnancy had antibodies to *M. hominis*. However, it is unclear whether exposure to *M. hominis* predated the occurrence of EP in these women. Further studies that simultaneously adjust for exposure to these organisms in women with EP would add substantially to our understanding of the pathogenic role each of these organisms play in EP.

The role of anaerobes (*Bacteroides* sp., *Peptococcus* sp., in particular) in PID has been largely restricted to reports of isolation rates. While it is possible to provoke antibody response to these organisms, there have been no studies that have associated long-term PID sequelae with a previously confirmed pelvic infection with these anaerobes.

Concurrent Infection and EP

Although there has been ample evidence for past infection with PID organisms demonstrated among EP cases, it has been rarely reported that these organisms were recovered from the affected tube, contralateral tube, or other sites. However, one report indicates that *C. trachomatis* may be recovered. Berenson and colleagues reported 6/27 EP cases as tubal culture-positive for *C. trachomatis*.[70] Whether this indicates anything more than a coincident finding, however, is debatable, because it is more likely that the etiology of EP is related to occlusion due to past infection rather than concurrent infection and inflammatory processes. Similar issues of the role of concurrent tubal infection have been raised with respect to TFI above.

Chronic Pelvic Pain and Recurrence of PID

The cause of chronic pelvic pain after PID can usually be traced to the presence of pelvic adhesions surrounding the fallopian tubes and ovaries. Falk first recognized this sequela in 17% of a series of post-PID patients.[11] This proportion was close to that reported later by Weström and colleagues in the Swedish follow-up studies (18.1% of post-PID patients versus 5% in controls).[21,22] Sixty-three percent of those with chronic pelvic pain were also infertile.

The retrospective cohort study of PID patients by Safrin and colleagues[25] also found that chronic pelvic pain for 6 months or more was reported by 24% of respondents and was significantly related to history of PID prior to admission. Recurrence of PID was reported by 43% of cases, occurring at a median of 2.1 months post-PID admission.

In the other large-scale follow-up study of hospitalized PID cases, Buchan and colleagues[55] reported that in comparison with hospitalized controls, the PID cases were ten times more likely to be admitted later for abdominal pain, four times more likely for gynecological pain, four times more likely for endometriosis, and eight times more likely for hysterectomy, an outcome not noted before in the literature.

Factors that Modify the Risk of PID Sequelae

Type of Organism

Investigators have observed that the different PID organisms are associated with a spectrum of clinical presentations. Gonococcal PID tends to present with symptoms that are more severe, and earlier than in the case of chlamydial PID. Chlamydial PID is often milder in presentation or even asymptomatic as suggested by the serological studies discussed above. This difference leads to a longer time period before treatment thereby allowing a clinically milder chlamydial infection in the tubes to cause more extensive structural damage. Thus, differences in PID etiology will ultimately affect the time interval before detection, diagnosis and treatment, as well as the risk of developing PID sequelae. The Swedish follow-up studies, which distinguished between PID associated with different organisms, found that women with nongonococcal PID had a 2.8-fold increased risk of TFI compared with those who had gonococcal PID.

Last, it has been noted that differences in the geographical distribution of these organisms may account for different results from epidemiological studies of factors relating to various PID sequelae. Thus, while the studies from the Scandinavian countries appeared to have a greater proportion of gonococcal, in-patient PID cases, reports from the United States tend to find a greater role for nongonococcal, chlamydial PID cases that are treated on an out-patient basis.

In addition, over the past two decades, there is a temporal difference in the occurrence of gonococcal versus nongonococcal PID. The earlier studies of PID and sequelae reported higher rates of gonococcal isolation, which later decreased. Coincident with the decrease in gonococcal infection were increases in the chlamydial infection rate.

Contraception

Another factor that appears to be associated with severity of PID is the type of contraceptive used at the time of PID diagnosis. Considerable debate has focused on the use of IUD and OCs versus barrier methods or no method and whether any of these can modify risk for PID.

Intrauterine Device (IUD) Use

The question of whether IUDs in general, or specific IUD types are more likely to cause PID and its sequelae has fueled considerable debate over its future use,[71-73] particularly in younger, nulligravid women. Past studies of IUD users and PID have been criticized for design flaws involving case definition and detection, appropriate control groups (non-IUD users, users of other methods of contraceptives), controlling for number of sexual partners, presence of STDs, sample size, and conclusions drawn from statistical test results. Presumably, any increased risk of TFI and EP associated with the IUD would be due to the occurrence of PID while the device was in situ. Two well-designed studies,[74-76] including a re-analysis of one, have looked at IUD use and TFI and determined that prior IUD use is associated with a two-(Lippes Loop) to sixfold (Dalkon Shield™) increase in risk of TFI when compared to non-IUD use. Similar conclusions of increased risk for EP have been made: prior use of the IUD and current use of the IUD are independently associated with an increased risk of EP.[48]

Oral Contraception

Several prevalence studies of PID found that OC use was less commonly reported among cases than controls, leading researchers to conclude that OC use might confer some protection against PID. For example, the Swedish studies[21-22,77-78] found that women who were OC users had a laparoscopically milder PID than women who either used other methods or no methods. Further, they reported that OC users were also less likely to have TFI (3.7%) than users of other methods (8.7% to 10.5%) and those using no method (11.8%). The authors did not have any information, however, on contraceptive use after the index laparoscopy in these follow-up studies. It has become clear in a review of these studies that the claim of a protective effect is limited by several study design issues. Washington and colleagues[79] pointed out that these initial studies (1) were limited to hospitalized cases of PID, representing less than 25% of all cases, and likely to be clinically severe in presentation, and (2) did not distinguish between gonococcal versus nongonococcal PID. Thus, the claim for a protective effect of OC use is at present limited to gonococcal PID, which is clinically more severe in presentation than is the case with chlamydial PID. Indeed, OC use may not protect against, and could even promote chlamydial PID due to OC enhancement of the cervical ectropion, thereby increasing susceptibility to *C. trachomatis* infection.

Resolution of this issue is critical for its potential impact on future prevention of PID and its sequelae. Specifically, recommendations have been made in favor of OC use for the purpose of preventing an initial episode or further recurrence of PID in women who are delaying childbearing. However, because of the possibility that OC use may actually promote unrecognized chlamydial PID (if symptoms are milder), the subsequent increased risk of chlamydia-associated tubal pathology and infertility should argue against this recommendation until further studies have been done specifically to address this issue.

Age

The effect of age at PID diagnosis has been discussed by Weström and colleagues in the longitudinal analysis of the Swedish data. Although younger (<25 years) women had a lower rate of infertility overall, than older women (25–35 years), the difference was due to a threefold increase in EP in the older group. The occurrence of TFI was equal in both age groups, however.

Timing of Diagnosis and Treatment for PID

There is evidence that the timing of diagnosis and treatment for PID can affect the risk of long-term sequelae. In a retrospective cohort study of women with one episode of laparoscopically diagnosed PID, delay in care of more than 2 days after the onset of PID symptoms was associated in a tripling of the risk for infertility or EP.[80] This has implications for the even greater risk of sequelae associated with undetected or silent PID. Because chlamydial PID in particular, tends to be associated with mild or absence of symptoms, the infection is not detected and women are not treated early in the disease. Thus, the risk of sequelae associated with this infection would be significantly increased by this delay in detection.

Douching Behavior

Recent reports of douching as a risk factor for PID[81–86] also have stimulated study into its role in PID sequelae related to fertility. Although the reports indicating a higher prevalence of douching among PID cases versus controls are consistent in their findings, this has not been the case with PID sequelae reports. While two case-control studies of ectopic pregnancy have identified douching to increase EP risk,[60,85] one report has found the opposite.[63] Future studies of douching and PID sequelae will have to take into consideration the presence of PID-associated organisms in the lower genital tract, and specific aspects of douching behavior (frequency, type of solution, timing during the menstrual cycle, and reason).[86]

Animal Models of PID Sequelae

Although it is possible from the studies described above to establish a clear relationship between PID and TFI and EP sequelae, there is still minimal knowledge about the pathogenesis of PID sequelae. The demonstration of infertility as an outcome after inoculation with organisms associated with PID (especially *C. trachomatis*) in various animal models has provided more information regarding the pathogenesis of PID sequelae such as TFI and EP. Several studies have reported successful efforts to simulate salpingitis in the mouse by inoculation of the mouse pneumonitis (MoPn) biovar of *C. trachomatis* into the ovarian bursa or uterine horn. Swenson and colleagues[87-88] were able to demonstrate not only the development of inflammatory exudate and hydrosalpinx, but also the significant occurrence of infertility. Tuffrey and colleagues also observed lower fertility in progesterone-treated inbred mice which were inoculated with human strains of *C. trachomatis*.[89] In both models, the infertility was due probably to the oviductal pathology caused by the infection. Three inbred mice strains inoculated intravaginally with MoPn also had significant decreases in fertility.[90]

Further work to elucidate the pathogenesis of PID sequelae has been done with pig-tailed monkeys by Patton and colleagues.[91] This group developed the "pocket model" in which live *C. trachomatis* organisms were inoculated into subcutaneous pockets containing salpingeal autotransplants. Subsequent inflammatory responses simulate the in situ model of salpingitis and a delayed hypersensitivity reaction can be further demonstrated by the injection of *C. trachomatis* HSP60 into these pockets. The pathogenesis of TFI has been suggested to be the result of tissue damage from immunopathologic reaction induced (specifically HSP60) chronic or repeat infections.

Future Research Issues

The evidence supporting PID as a major risk factor for tubal infertility, ectopic pregnancy, and chronic pelvic pain is abundant. To reduce the incidence of these sequelae, the incidence of PID must be reduced. This can be accomplished by reducing the reservoir of sexually transmitted pathogens, and asymptomatic PID. Because most asymptomatic PID is associated with chlamydial infection, it is ultimately, the reduction of the chlamydial infection reservoir that should be addressed.

Reduction of the reservoir of chlamydial infection involves, (1) identification of appropriate diagnosis and treatment of symptomatic patients, (2) screening of high-risk populations to identify asymptomatic infections, (3) identification and testing of exposed sexual contacts, and (4) treatment with antibiotic therapy effective against chlamydial infection.[92,93] By reduction of asymptomatic chlamydial infections, the reduction of asymptomatic PID and its sequelae is possible.

Future research can augment efforts at the reduction of the chlamydial infection reservoir in the specific areas outlined above. To better characterize high-risk populations, behavioral risk factors for chlamydial infection may be identified for both partners. More complete ascertainment of asymptomatic cases will be possible using amplified DNA technology (PCR and LCR). The latter two improvements will also improve identification and testing of sexual contacts. Last, the more widespread use of single-dose antibiotic therapy will improve treatment compliance.

Clearly, these efforts to more effectively reduce the reservior of infections will come at a cost. Not every community will have access to the most effective screening technologies to identify cases. But, where the resources exist to reduce this reservoir, the cost-effectiveness of the measures taken will be evident. The cost of screening and treating asymptomatic cases of PID will be far less than the cost of treating tubal infertility, ectopic pregnancy, and chronic pelvic pain.

References

1. Noeggerath E. Latent gonorrhea, especially with regard to its influence on fertility in women. *Transactions of the American Gynecologic Society* 1877; **1**:268–293.
2. Mardh P-A. Pelvic inflammatory disease and related disorders; novel observations. *Scand J Obstet Gynecol* 1990;**69**(suppl):83–87.
3. Weström L, Wølner-Hanssen P. Pathogenesis of pelvic inflammatory disease. *Genitourin Med* 1993;**69**:9–17.
4. McCormack WM. Pelvic inflammatory disease. *N Engl J Med* 1994;**330**(2): 115–119.
5. Wølner-Hanssen P, Kiviat NK, Holmes KK. Atypical pelvic inflammatory disease: Subacute, chronic or subclinical upper genital tract infection in women, in Holmes KK, Mardh P-A, Sparling PF, Wiesner PJ. (eds): *Sexually transmitted disease*, 2nd ed. New York, McGraw-Hill, 1990,615–620.
6. Washington AE, Katz P. Cost and payment source for pelvic inflammatory disease. Trends and projections, 1983 through 2000. *J Am Med Assoc* 1991; **266**(18):2565–2569.
7. Mosher WD, Aral SO. Factors related to infertility in the United States 1965–1976. *Sex Trans Dis* 1985;**12**:117–123.
8. Cates W, Rolfs RT, Aral SO. Sexually transmitted diseases, pelvic inflammatory disease, and infertility: An epidemiologic update. *Epidemiol Rev* 1990;**12**: 199–220.
9. Holtz F. Klinische Studien uber die nicht tuberculose Salpingo-phoritis. *Acta Obstetrica et Gynecologica Scandinavica* 1930;**10**(suppl).
10. Hedberg E, Speyz S. Acute salpingitis. View on prognosis and treatment *Acta Obstetrica and Gynecologica Scandinavica* 1958;**37**:131–154.
11. Falk V. Treatment of acute non-tuberculous salpingitis with antibiotics alone and in combination with glucocorticoids. *Acta Obstetrica et Gynecologica Scandinavica* 1965;**44**(suppl 6).

12. Krook G, Juhlin I. Problems in diagnosis, treatment and control of gonorrheal infections. *Acta Derm Venereol (Stockh)* 1965;**45**:242.

13. Henry-Suchet J, Catalan F, Loffredo V, et al. Microbiology of specimens obtained by laparoscopy from controls and from patients with pelvic inflammatory disease of infertility. *Am J Obstet Gynecol* 1980;**7**.

14. Henry-Suchet J, Catalan F, Loffredo V, Sanson MJ, Debache C, Pigeau F. *Chlamydia trachomatis* associated with chronic inflammation in abdominal specimens from women selected for tuboplasty. *Fertil Steril* 1981;**36**:599–605.

15. Henry-Suchet J, Utzmann C, De Brux JEJ, Ardoin P, Catalan F. Microbiologic study of chronic inflammation associated with tubal factor infertility: Role of *Chlamydia trachomatis*. *Fertil Steril* 1987;**47**:274–277.

16. Henry-Suchet J. *Chlamydia trachomatis* infection and infertility in women. *J Reprod Med* 1988;**91**:912–914.

17. Shepherd MK, Jones RB. Recovery of *Chlamydia trachomatis* from endometrial and fallopian tube biopsies in women with infertility of tubal origin. *Fertil Steril* 1989;**52**:232–238.

18. Thejls H, Gnarpe J, Lundqvist O, Heimer G, Larsson G, Victor A. Diagnosis and prevalence of persistent *Chlamydia* infection in infertile women: tissue culture, direct antigen detection, and serology. *Fertil Steril* 1992;**55**: 304–310.

19. Campbell LA, Patton DL, Moore DE, Cappuccio AL, Mueller BA, Wang SP. Detection of *Chlamydia trachomatis* deoxyribonucleic acid in women with tubal infertility. *Fertil Steril* 1991;**59**(1):45–50.

20. Patton DL, Cosgrove-Sweeney YT, Plier PK, Burczak JD, Clark AM, Lee HH, Stamm WE. Detection of *Chlamydia trachomatis* by cell culture, polymerase chain reaction (PCR) and ligase chain reaction (LCR) in upper and lower tract reproductive tissues in an experimental monkey model of PID, in Orfila J, Byrne GI, Chernesky MA, Grayston JT, Jones RB, Ridgway GL, Saikku P, Schachter J, Stamm WE, Stephens RS (eds): *Chlamydial Infections*. Bologna, Italy, Societa Editrice Esculapio, 1994, pp 314–317

21. Weström L. Incidence, prevalence, and trends of acute pelvic inflammatory disease and its consequences in industrialized countries. *Am J Obstet Gynecol* 1980;**138**:880–892.

22. Weström L, Joesoef MJ, Reynolds G, Hagdu A, Thompson SE. Pelvic inflammatory disease and fertility: A cohort study of 1844 women with laparoscopically verified disease and 657 control women with normal laparoscopic results. *Sex Trans Dis* 1992;**19**(4):185–192.

23. Weström L. Sexually transmitted diseases and infertility. *Sex Trans Dis* 1994;**21**(suppl):S32–S37.

24. Adler A. Trends for gonorrhoeae and pelvic inflammatory disease in England and Wales and for gonorrhea in a defined population. *Am J Obstet Gynecol* 1980;**138**:901–904.

25. Safrin S, Schachter J, Dahrouge D, Sweet RL. Long-term sequelae of acute pelvic inflammatory disease: A retrospective cohort study. *Am J Obstet Gynecol* 1992;**166**:1300–1305.

26. Punnonen R, Terho P, Nikkanen V, Meurman O. Chlamydial serology in infertile women by immunofluoresence. *Fertil Steril* 1979;**31**:656–659.

27. Cevenini R, Possati G, La Placa M. *Chlamydia trachomatis* infection in infertile women, in Mardh P-A, Holmes KK, Oriel D, Piot P, Schachter J (eds): *Chlamydial Infections*. Amsterdam, Elsevier Biomedical Press, 1982, pp 189–192.

28. Jones RB, Ardery BR, Hui SL, Cleary RE. Correlation between serum antichlamydial antibodies and tubal factor as a cause of infertility. *Fertil Steril* 1982;**38**:553–558.

29. Moore DE, Foy H, Daling JR. Increased frequency of serum antibodies to *Chlamydia trachomatis* in infertility due to tubal disease. *Lancet* 1982;**ii**: 574–577.

30. Gump DW, Gibson M, Ashikaga T. Evidence of prior pelvic inflammatory disease and its relationship to *Chlamydia trachomatis* antibody and intrauterine contraceptive device. *Am J Obstet Gynecol* 1983;**146**:153–159.

31. Svensson L, Mardh P-A, Weström L. Infertility after acute salpingitis with special reference to *Chlamydia trachomatis. Fertil Steril* 1983;**40**:322–329.

32. Conway D, Caul EO, Hull MGR, et al. Chlamydial serology in fertile and infertile women. *Lancet* 1984;**i**:191–193.

33. Sellors JW, Mahony JB, Chernesky MA, Rath DJ. Tubal factor infertility: An association with prior chlamydial infection and asymptomatic salpingitis. *Fertil Steril* 1988;**49**:451–457.

34. Bjercke S, Purvis K. Chlamydial serology in the investigation of infertility. *Hum Reprod* 1992;**7**:621–624.

35. Reniers J, Collet M, Frost E, Leclerc A, Ivanoff B, Meheus A. Chlamydial antibodies and tubal infertility. *Int J Epidemiol* 1989;**18**(1):261–263.

36. Morrison RP. Chlamydial hsp60 and the immunopathogenesis of chlamydial disease. *Semin Immunol* 1991;**3**(1):25–33.

37. Toye B, Laferriere C, Claman P, Jessamine P, Peeling RW. Association between antibody to the *Chlamydial* heat shock protein and tubal infertility. *J Infect Dis* 1993;**168**:1236–1240.

38. Mueller BA, Luz-Jimenez M, Daling JR, Moore DE, McKnight B, Weiss NS. Risk factors for tubal infertility. Influence of history of prior pelvic inflammatory disease. *Sex Trans Dis* 1992;**19**(1):28–34.

39. Cates W, Wasserheit JN. Genital chlamydial infections: Epidemiology and reproductive sequelae. *Am J Obstet Gynecol* 1991;**164**:1771–1781.

40. Mabey DC, Ogbaselassie G, Robertson JN, Heckels JE, Ward ME. Tubal infertility in the Gambia: Chlamydial and gonococcal serology in women with tubal occlusion compared with pregnant controls. *Bull WHO* 1985;**63**(6): 1107–1113.

41. Tjam KH, Zeilmaker GH, Alberda ATh, van Heijst BYM, de Roo JC, Polak-Vogelzang AA, va Joost Th, Stolz E, Michel MF. Prevalence of antibodies to *Chlamydia trachomatis, Neisseria gonorrhoeae,* and *Mycoplasma hominis* in infertile women. *Genitourin Med* 1985;**61**:175–178.

42. Robertson JN, Ward ME, Conway D, Caul EO. Chlamydial and gonococcal antibodies in sera of infertile women with tubal obstruction. *J Clin Pathol* 1987;**40**:377–383.

43. Collet M, Reniers J, Frost E, Gass R, Yvert F, Leclerc A, Roth-Meyer C, Ivanoff B, Meheus A. Infertility in Central Africa: Infection is the cause. *Int J Gynecol Obstet* 1988;**26**(3):423–428.

44. De Muylder X, Laga M, Tennstedt C, Van Dyck E, Aelbers GN, Piot P. The role of *Neisseria gonorrhoeae* and *Chlamydia trachomatis* in pelvic inflammatory disease and its sequelae in Zimbabwe. *J Infect Dis* 1990;**162**(2):501–505.

45. Miettinen A, Heinonnen PK, Teisala K, Hakkarainen K, Punnonen R. Serologic evidence for the role of *Chlamydia trachomatis, Neisseria gonorrhoeae,* and

Mycoplasma hominis in the etiology of tubal factor infertility and ectopic pregnancy. *Sex Trans Dis* 1990;**17**(1):10–14.

46. Møller BR, Taylor-Robinson DA, Furr PM, Toft B, Allen J. Serologic evidence that chlamydiae and mycoplasmas are involved in infertility of women. *J Reprod Fert* 1985;**73**:237–240.

47. Weström L, Bengtsson LP, Mardh P-A. Incidence, trends and risk of ectopic pregnancy in a population of women. *Br J Obstet Gynecol* 1981;**82**:15–18.

48. Chow WH, Daling JR, Cates W Jr, Greenberg RS. Epidemiology of ectopic pregnancy. *Epidemiol Rev* 1987;**9**:70–94.

49. Marchbanks PA, Annegers JF, Coulam CB, Strathy NH, Kurland LT. Risk factors for ectopic pregnancy. A population-based study. *JAMA* 1988;**259**: 823–827.

50. Hadgu A, Weström L, Johnson R, Koch G. Analysis of a longitudinal ectopic pregnancy data set from Lund, Sweden. Presented at the 10th meeting of the International Society for Sexually Transmitted Disease Research, 1993, Helsinki, Finland.

51. Coste J, Job-Spira N, Aublet-Cuvelier B, Germain E, Glowaczower E, Fernandez H, Pouly JL. Incidence of ectopic pregnancy. First results of a population-based register in France. *Human Reprod* 1994;**9**(4):742–745.

52. Coste J, Laumon B, Bremond A, Collet P, Job-Spira N. Sexually transmitted diseases as major causes of ectopic pregnancy: Results from a large case-control study in France. *Fertil Steril* 1994;**62**(2):289–295.

53. Goldner TE, Lawson HW, Xie Z, Atrash HK. Surveillance for ectopic pregnancy—United States, 1970–1989. *MMWR CDC Surv Summ* 1993;**42**(SS-6): 73–85.

54. Hillis S, Harms L, Marchbanks P, Amsterdam L, MacKenzie W. Recurrent *Chlamydia* infections as a risk factor for ectopic pregnancy, in Orfila J, Byrne GI, Chernesky MA, Grayston JT, Jones RB, Ridgway GL, Saikku P, Schachter J, Stamm WE, Stephens RS (eds): *Chlamydial Infections*. Societa Editrice Esculapio, Bologna, Italy, 1994, pp 611–613.

55. Buchan H, Vessey M, Goldacre M, Fairweather J. Morbidity following pelvic inflammatory disease. *Br J Obstet Gynecol* 1993;**100**(6):558–562.

56. Svensson L, Mardh P-A, Ahlgren M, Nordenskjold F. Ectopic pregnancy and antibodies to *Chlamydia trachomatis*. *Fertil Steril* 1985;**44**:313–317.

57. Brunham RC, Binns B, McDowell J, Paraskevas M. *Chlamydia trachomatis* infection in women with ectopic pregnancy. *Obstet Gynecol* 1986;**67**: 722–726.

58. Walters MD, Eddy CA, Gibbs RS, Schachter J, Holden AEC, Pauerstein CJ. Antibodies to *Chlamydia trachomatis* and ectopic pregnancy. *Am J Obstet Gynecol* 1988;**259**:1823–1827.

59. Chaim W, Sarov B, Sarov I, Piura B, Cohen A, Insler V. Serum IgG and IgA antibodies to *Chlamydia* in ectopic pregnancies. *Contraception* 1989;**40**: 59–71.

60. Chow JM, Yonekura ML, Richwald GA, Greenland S, Sweet RL, Schachter J. The association between *Chlamydia trachomatis* and ectopic pregnancy: A matched-pair case-control study. *JAMA* 1990;**263**:3164–3167.

61. Coste J, Job-Spira N, Fernandez H, Papiernik E, Spira A. Risk factors for ectopic pregnancy: A case-control study in France, with special focus on infectious factors. *Am J Epidemiol* 1991;**133**(9):839–849.

62. Brunham RC, Peeling R, Maclean I, Kosseim ML, Paraskevas M. *Chlamydia trachomatis*-associated ectopic pregnancy: Serologic and histologic correlates. *J Infect Dis* 1992;**165**(6):1076–1081.
63. Phillips RS, Tuomala RE, Feldblum PJ, Schachter J, Rosenberg MJ, Aronson MJ. The effect of cigarette smoking, *Chlamydia trachomatis* infections, and vaginal douching on ectopic pregnancy. *Obstet Gynecol* 1992;**79**(1):85–90.
64. Sheffield PA, Moore DE, Voigt LF, Scholes D, Wang SP, Grayston JT, Daling JR. The association between *Chlamydia trachomatis* serology and pelvic damage in women with tubal ectopic gestations. *Fertil Steril* 1993;**60**(6):970–975.
65. Odland JO, Anestad G, Rasmussen S, Lundgren R, Dalaker K. Ectopic pregnancy and chlamydial serology. *Int J Obstet Gynecol* 1993;**43**(3):271–275.
66. Wagar EA, Schachter J, Bavoil P, Stephens RS. Differential human serologic response to two 60,000 molecular weight *Chlamydia trachomatis* antigens. *J Infect Dis* 1990;**162**:992–997.
67. Robertson JN, Hogston P, Ward ME. Gonococcal and chlamydial antibodies in ectopic and intrauterine pregnancy. *Br J Obstet Gynecol* 1988;**95**(7): 711–716.
68. Ville Y, Leruez M, Glowaczower E, Robertson JN, Ward ME. The role of *Chlamydia trachomatis* and *Neisseria gonorrhoeae* in the aetiology of ectopic pregnancy in Gabon. *Br J Obstet Gynecol* 1991;**98**(12):1260–1266.
69. Miettinen A, Paavonen J, Jansson E, Leinikki P. Enzyme immunoassay for serum antibody to *Mycoplasma hominis* in women with acute pelvic inflammatory disease. *Sex Transm Dis* 1983;**10**:289–293.
70. Berenson A, Hammill H, Martens M, Faro S. Bacteriologic findings with ectopic pregnancy. *J Reprod Med* 1991;**36**:118–120.
71. Aral SO, Mosher WD, Cates W Jr. Contraceptive use, pelvic inflammatory disease, and fertility problems among American women. *Am J Obstet Gynecol* 1987;**157**:59–64.
72. Eschenbach D. Earth, motherhood, and the intrauterine device. *Fertil Steril* 1992;**57**(6):1177–1179.
73. Grimes DA. The intrauterine device, pelvic inflammatory disease, and infertility: The confusion between hypothesis and knowledge. *Fertil Steril* 1992;**58**(4):670–673.
74. Daling JR, Weiss NS, Metch BJ, Chow WH, Soderstrom RM, Moore DE, et al. Primary tubal infertility in relation to the use of an intrauterine device. *N Engl J Med* 1985;**312**:937–941.
75. Cramer DW, Schiff I, Schoenbaum SC, Gibson M, Belisle S, Albrecht B, et al. Tubal infertility and the intrauterine device. *N Engl J Med* 1985;**312**: 941–947.
76. Daling JR, Weiss NS, Voight LF, McKnight B, Moore DE. The intrauterine device and primary tubal infertility. *N Engl J Med* 1992;**326**(3):203–204.
77. Wølner-Hanssen P. Oral contraceptive use modifies the manifestations of pelvic inflammatory disease. *Br J Obstet Gynecol* 1986;**93**:619–624.
78. Wølner-Hanssen P, Eschenbach DA, Paavonen J, et al. Decreased risk of symptomatic chlamydial pelvic inflammatory disease associated with oral contraceptive use. *JAMA* 1990;**263**:54–59.
79. Washington AE, Gove S, Schachter J, Sweet RL. Oral contraceptives, *Chlamydia trachomatis* infection and pelvic inflammatory disease. *JAMA* 1985; **253**:2246–2250.

80. Hillis SD, Riduan J, Marchbanks PA, Wasserheit JN, Cates W, Weström L. Delayed care of pelvic inflammatory disease as a risk factor for impaired fertility. *Am J Obstet Gynecol* 1993;**168**(5):1503–1509.

81. Neumann HH, DeCherney A. Douching and pelvic inflammatory disease. *N Engl J Med* 1976;**295**:789.

82. Forrest KA, Washington AE, Daling JR, Sweet RL. Vaginal douching as a potential risk factor for pelvic inflammatory disease. *J Natl Med Assoc* 1989; **89**:159–165.

83. Wølner-Hanssen P, Eschenbach DA, Paavonen J, Kiviat N, Stevens C, Koutsky L, DeRouen T, Critchlow C, Holmes KK. Association between vaginal douching and pelvic inflammatory disease. *JAMA* 1990;**263**:1926–1941.

84. Meyer L, Soulat C. Vaginal douching and ectopic pregnancy. *JAMA* 1991; **265**:2670–2671.

85. Daling JR, Weiss NS, Schwartz SM, Stergachis A, Wang SP, Foy H, Chu J, McKnight B, Grayston JT. Vaginal douching and the risk of tubal pregnancy. *Epidemiol* 1991;**2**:40–48.

86. Schachter J, Chow JM. Vaginal douching as it relates to reproductive health complications. *Curr Opin Infect Dis* 1993;**6**:27–30.

87. Swenson CE, Schachter J. Infertility as a consequence of chlamydial infection of the upper genital tract in female mice. *Sex Trans Dis* 1984;**11**(2):64–67.

88. Tuffrey M, Alexander F, Inman C, Ward M. Correlation of infertility with altered tubal morphology and function in mice with salpingitis induced by a human genital-tract isolate of *Chlamydia trachomatis. J Reprod Fertil* 1990;**88**:295–305.

89. Swenson CE, Donegan E, Schachter J. *Chlamydia trachomatis*-induced salpingitis in mice. *J Infect Dis* 1983;**148**(6):1101–1107.

90. de la Maza LM, Pal S, Khamesipour A, Peterson E. Intravaginal inoculation of mice with Chlamydia trachomatis mouse pneumonitis biovar results in infertility. *Infect Immun* 1994;**62**(5):2094–2097.

91. Patton DL, Cosgrove-Sweeney YT, Kuo C-C. Demonstration of delayed hypersensitivity in *Chlamydia trachomatis* salpingitis in monkeys: A pathologic mechanism of tubal damage. *J Infect Dis* 1994;**169**:680–683.

92. World Health Organization. Infections, pregnancies and infertility: Perspectives on prevention. *Fertil Steril* 1987;**47**:964–968.

93. Centers for Disease Control. 1993 Sexually Transmitted Diseases Treatment Guidelines. *MMWR* 1993;**42**(No RR-14):47–81.

12
Histopathology of Genital Tract Infection with *C. trachomatis* and *N. gonorrhoeae*

Nancy Kiviat

Over the last 2 decades, a great deal has been learned about the molecular biology and the clinical manifestations of *Chlamydia trachomatis* and *Neisseria gonorrhoeae*. Relatively few studies, however, have focused on the histopathological changes induced by the agents in the endocervix, endometrium, or fallopian tubes. Our understanding of the tissue changes resulting from infection with these agents has been derived from a small number of animal studies, organ culture studies, and studies of women presenting with suspected pelvic inflammatory disease (PID).

Observations in Animal and Organ Culture Systems

C. trachomatis

Several animal models for *C. trachomatis* genital tract infection have been developed, including ones in which the organism is inoculated either into the uterus or directly into the fallopian tubes[1-5] of experimental animals. Although endometrial infection appears to be possible using such systems, detailed descriptions of the histopathological changes with endometrial infection in such animals systems have not appeared. Most studies using this approach have focused almost exclusively on changes within the fallopian tubes or fimbrial tissues. Another model for the study of salpingitis, described by Patton and colleagues, includes rhesus and pigtailed monkeys, in which tissue biopsies of the salpinx and fimbria are autotransplanted to the subcutaneous abdominal skin. The resulting subcutaneous pockets (containing the pieces of fimbrial tissue) are then inoculated with *C. trachomatis*. This model has the advantage of allowing the investigator to repeatedly obtain tissue samples over time in a relatively easy manner. The most complete descriptions of the sequential histologic changes with primary and repeated infection of tubal tissue (fimbriae) have utilized this subcutaneous pocket model.[6,7] With primary infection, fimbrial subepithelial tissues were noted to be infiltrated with polymorphonuclear cells (PMNs) by the second day after inoculation, with a dense infiltrate of lymphocytes and plasma cells noted throughout the tissue by day 3 or 4. In addition, at this time, lymphocytes were seen migrating into the overlying epithelium, especially in areas where damaged vacuolated epithelial cells were present. Luminal erthrocytes, lymphocytes, and desquamated epithelial cells were also noted. This picture persisted through day 14. By day 21 only minimal inflammation remained. When animals were later reinfected with the organism, the histologic findings differed from those seen with primary infection in that a mixed mononuclear-PMN infiltrate clustering in the submucosal regions and migrating into the overlying damaged epithelium was seen by day 2 or 3. By day 7, lymphoid "follicle-like" clusters appears with an increase in the number of plasma cells noted in the submucosa. Less epithelial cell damage appeared present at this time. Similar, but more intense changes accompanied by extensive deep stromal tissue fibrosis was noted when the animals were reinfected a third time.[6,7] Hydrosalpinx formation following *C. trachomatis* infection is not uncommon. During acute tubal infection, histologic findings are similar to those that have been described in endometrial infection.

N. gonorrhoeae

In situ animal models for *N. gonorrhoeae* infection have not been developed and experimental infection is limited to organ culture system.[9] Studies using such systems have demonstrated that pili and other surface proteins initially aid attachment of the organism to nonciliated epithelial cells. The cilia on adjacent cells appear to be impaired by gonococcal lipooligosaccharaide (endotoxin), perhaps resulting in increased susceptibility to subsequent organism attachment and cell death. In any case the organisms are soon noted in the subepithelial area. This process evokes a dense infiltrate of PMN leukocytic response in the subepithelial area, with PMNs also seen moving through the overlying sloughing epithelium.[10,11]

Histopathological Changes with *C. trachomatis* and/or *N. gonorrhoeae* Infection of the Human Female Genital Tract

Surprisingly, only recently has there been any attempt to correlate specific histologic changes seen in the endocervix, endometrium, or fallopian tubes with infection by specific organisms. Studies of tissue changes induced by *C. trachomatis* or *N. gonorrhoeae* infection of the human female genital tract are complicated by the fact that there is some disagreement as to what cells are normally present at this site. A variety of inflammatory cells are commonly found in the endocervix, endometrial, and fallopian tube submucosal regions. In addition to the presence of lymphocytes and PMNs during menstruation, pathologists have long appreciated the fact that normally several days prior to the regular sloughing of the endometrium, lymphocytes are present within the endometrium.[12] Likewise, a scattering of lymphocytes are frequently seen in the cervix, endocervix, and fallopian tubes, and such changes are considered normal. Whether denser lymphocytic infiltrates, lymphoid follicles, or even scattered plasma cells are normal at such sites or represent evidence of present subclinical or past infection, is controversial. Some investigators state that such findings are self-limited and resolve without antibiotic therapy, while others make a histologic diagnosis of chronic endocervicitis and endometritis on the basis of such findings. At least one group has reported that lymphoid follicles were associated with positive *C. trachomatis* serology.[13] Studies focusing on such changes in which more sensitive methods (such as PCR) are used for identification of specific pathogens may help resolve such issues in the future.

Endocervicitis

A number of studies have examined the histopathology of endocervicitis caused by *C. trachomatis*.[14-17] Most such studies have reported finding changes similar to those seen in trachoma to be present.[18] Dense infiltrates of plasma cells and lymphocytes with lymphoid follicles are most frequently mentioned. Unfortunately, most of these studies either did not include culture confirmation of *C. trachomatis* or lacked comprehensive cultures for other pathogens. One recent study compared endocervical biopsies from women with suspected endocervical infection (including 32 women seen in a sexually transmitted disease [STD] clinic with suspected cervicitis and 27 women with suspected acute salpingitis) to those of women without clinical or laboratory evidence of infection.[15] All participants were cultured for *C. trachomatis*, *N. gonorrhoeae*, herpes simplex virus (HSV), and *T. vaginalis*. Histologic changes that were found to be associated with a positive culture for *C. trachomatis* included focal loss of surface columnar epithelium, but not with necrosis and destruction of the underlying tissue as was the case for the example in HSV infection. *Chlamydia trachomatis* was characterized by dense subepithelial plasma cell infiltrates with neutrophil infiltration of the columnar epithelium and germinal center formations that was generally periglandular in location. Lymphocytes, histocytes, and plasma cells were always present, with plasma cells generally greatly outnumbering other inflammatory cells. However, because this study was limited to women presenting to a STD clinic or a hospital emergency room with either suspected cervicitis and/or suspected upper genital tract infection, it is possible that the changes seen in this study represent only one end of the spectrum of cervicitis caused by *C. trachomatis* and that less severe changes are in fact common. These features are demonstrated in Figures

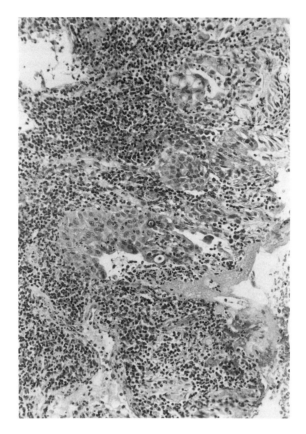

FIGURE 12.1. This section of endocervical tissue was first stained with monoclonal antibodies to *C. trachomatis* and then with hematoxylin and eosin (magnification ×4,000). Intraepithelial inclusions are seen, as well as intraepithelial polymorphonuclear leukocytes and underlying dense accumulations of lymphocytes and plasma cells.

12.1 to 12.3. Surprisingly, infection with *N. gonorrhoeae* was not associated with marked inflammation, and may have reflected the presence of focal disease with inadequate biopsy or patient selection bias.

Endometritis

Traditionally, the pathologists have classified endometritis as acute or chronic, with the diagnosis of acute endometritis being based on the presence of microabscesses or neutrophils filling and destroying endometrial glands, while chronic endometritis has been based on the presence of variable numbers of plasma cells within the endometrial stroma.[12,13,19] This terminology, which predated the isolation of *C. trachomatis* and our appreciation of the importance of this agent in the female upper genital tract

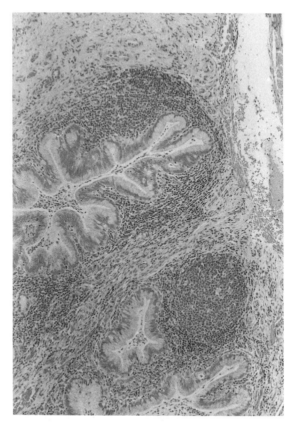

FIGURE 12.2. Chlamydial cervicitis with well-formed periglandular germinal centers.

infection, is confusing, as it is now known that the so-called chronic changes (such as the presence of dense infiltrates of plasma cells) appear within several days of initial infection. For this reason, such terminology is best avoided. Thus, Ingerslev and colleagues,[20] Mardh and coworkers,[21] Paavonen,[22] and Winkler and Crum[23–25] found PMNs and dense plasma cell infiltrates and a variety of other inflammatory changes such as edema, epithelial atypias, stromal necrosis, and lymphoid follicles in women with laboratory evidence of chlamydial infection. Winkler and Crum and Paavonen and coworkers classified the amount of inflammation present as mild, moderate, or severe and found that severe endometritis correlated best with evidence of *C. trachomatis* infection. Unfortunately, patients in all but the study by Paavonen did not have comprehensive analysis for other pathogens. In another study,[26] 69 consecutive women presenting with suspected acute PID underwent microbiological evaluation for upper genital tract infection, laparoscopic examination for evidence of salpingitis, and endometrial biopsy. *Chlamydia trachomatis* or *N. gonorrhoeae* was found in the upper genital tract of 90% (34 women) of those with proven upper

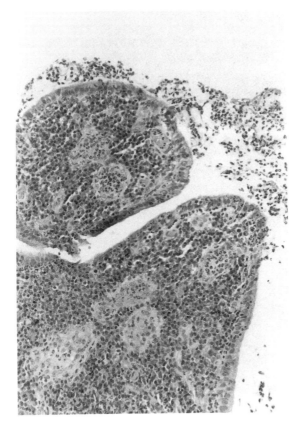

FIGURE 12.3. Endocervical biopsy showing focal loss of columnar cells, intraepithelial polymorphonuclear leukocytes, and dense underlying inflammation (plasma cells and lymphocytes).

genital tract infection. Comparing the endometrial histology of those with proven upper genital tract infection and laproscopically proven salpingitis to those with neither laboratory or laparascopic evidence of upper genital tract infection, the features that were associated with positive upper tract cultures and a laparoscopic diagnosis of salpingitis included intraluminal or any intraepithelial neutrophils, dense superficial stromal inflammation (defined as on average greater than 50 mononuclear cells per 400 × field), the presence of any number of plasma cells, and lymphoid aggregates containing transformed lymphocytes (Figures 12.4–12.6). The presence of both five or more neutrophils per 400 × field in the endometrial surface epithelium and one or more plasma cells per 120 × field within the endometrial stroma had a sensitivity of 92% and a specificity of 87% for the diagnosis of culture-proven upper genital tract infection and laparoscopically proven salpingitis. Immunofluorescence stains using monoclonal antibodies directed against *C. trachomatis* elementary bodies shows that the organism was located

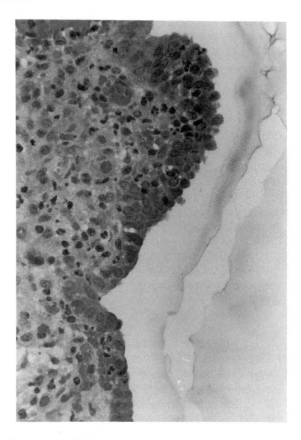

FIGURE 12.4. Endometrial biopsy: polymorphonuclear leukocytes within the surface epithelium with underlying dense inflammation of plasma cells and lymphocytes typical of culture-proven Chlamydial or gonococcal endometritis.

primarily in the surface epithelium. Differentiation of features associated with *C. trachomatis* versus *N. gonorrhoeae* was difficult, as only a minority of women had upper genital tract infection with one but not both of these agents. However, features that were associated with *C. trachomatis* as opposed to *N. gonorrhoeae* infection included a mean higher number of plasma cells and the presence of lymphoid follicles containing transformed lymphocytes. Tissue fragmentation was more often seen with *N. gonorrhoeae*. Examples of features associated with *C. trachomatis* and *N. gonorrhoeae* endometrial infection are shown in the figures.

Salpingitis

Animal models of *C. trachomatis* salpingitis as well as the few cases of microscopically examined laboratory confirmed *C. trachomatis* salpingitis in women that have been reported in the current literature demonstrate that the histologic changes observed vary with the stage of infection examined (i.e., days since innoculation of the organism in the fallopian tube). In addition, animal studies (summarized above) have shown that the sequence of histologic changes noted depend on whether previous infection has occurred. The inflammatory cellular infiltrate is similar to that seen in chlamydial and gonococcal endometritis described.[27] Early in infection, edema, dilation of capillaries, and a dense inflammatory infiltrate of lymphocytes, plasma cells, and PMNs occur. While this infiltrate is most dense in the submucosal area, it commonly extends into the adjacent muscle, and not infrequently onto the serosal surface. Polymorphonuclear cells also infiltrate the overlying tubal epithelium and the damaged epithelial cells are seen sloughing into the tubal lumen. Tubal wall fibrosis and the formation of hydrosalpinx may occur later.

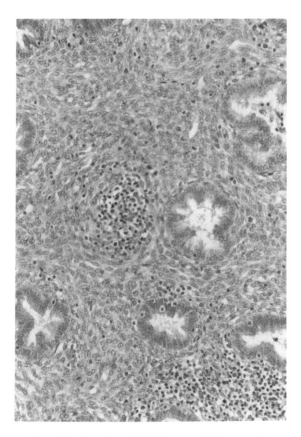

FIGURE 12.5. Periglandular lymphoid follicles containing transformed lymphocytes in an endometrial biopsy from a woman with Chlamydial endometritis.

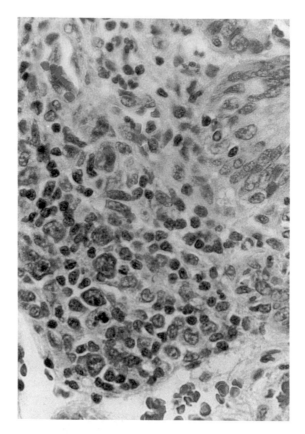

FIGURE 12.6. High-power view of endometritis showing a germinal center containing transformed lymphocytes.

References

1. Patton DL, Landers DV, Schachter J. Experimental *Chlamydia trachomatis* salpingitis in mice: Initial studies on the characterization of the leukocyte response to chlamydial infection. *JID* 1989;**159**:1105–1110.
2. Patton DL, Halbert SA, Kuo CC, Wang SP, Holmes KK. Host response to primary *Chlamydia trachomatis* infection of the fallopian tube in pig-tailed monkeys. *Fertil Steril* 1983;**40**:825–840.
3. Møller BR, Mardh P-A. Experimental salpingitis in Grivet monkeys by *Chlamydia trachomatis*. *Acta path microbiol Scand Sect B* 1980;**88**:107–114.
4. Patton DL, Halbert SA, Kuo C-C, Wang S-P, Holmes KK. Host response to primary Chlamydia trachomatis infection of the fallopian tube in pig-tailed monkeys. *Fertil Steril* 1983;**40**:825–840.

5. Barron AL, White HJ, Rank RG, Soloff. Target tissues associated with genital infection of female Guinea pigs by the Chlamydial agent of Guinea pig inclusion conjunctivitis. *JID* 1979;**139**:60–68.

6. Patton KL, Kuo CC, Wang SP, Brenner RM, Sternfeld MD, Morse SA, Barnes RC. Chlamydial infection of subcutaneous fimbrial transplants in cynomolgus and rhesus monkeys. *J Infect Dis* 1987;**155**:229–235.

7. Patton DL, Kuo C-C. Histopathology of *Chlamydia trachomatis* salpingitis after primary and repeated reinfections in the monkey subcutaneous pocket model. *J Reprod Fertil* 1980;**85**:647–656.

8. Patton DL, Kuo CC, Wang S-P, Halbert SA. Distal tubal obstruction induced by repeated *Chlamydia trachomatis* salpingeal infection in pig-tailed macaques. *J Infect Dis* 1987;**155**:1292–1299.

9. Shaw JH, Falkow S. Model for invasion of human tissue culture cells by *Neisseria gonorrhoeae*. *Infect Immun* 1988;**56**:1625–1632.

10. Pierce WA, Buchanan TM. Attachment role of gonococcal pili: Optimum conditions and quantitation of adherence of isolated pili to human cells in vitro. *J Clin Invest* 1978;**61**:131.

11. King GL, Swanson J. Studies on gonococcus infection: XV. Identification of surface proteins of *Neisseria gonorrhoeae* correlated with leukocyte association. *Infect Immun* 1978;**21**:575.

12. Kruman RJ, Mazur MT. Benign disease of the endometrium, in Blaustein A (ed): *Pathology of the Female Genital Tract*, 2nd ed. New York, Springer-Verlag, 1982, p 279.

13. Burke RK, Hertig AT, Miele CA. Prognostic value of subacute focal inflammation of the endometrium with special reference to pelvic adhesions as observed on laparoscopic examination. *J Reprod Med* 1985;**30**:646–650.

14. Hare MJ, Toone E. Taylor-Robinson D, et al. Follicular cervicitis: Colposcopic apearances and associations with *Chlamydia trachomatis*. *Br J Obstet Gynecol* 1981;**88**:174–180.

15. Kiviat NB, Paavonen JA, Wølner-Hanssen P, Critchlow CW, Stamm WE, Douglas J, Eschenbach DA, Corey LA, Holmes KK. Histopathology of endocervical infection caused by *Chlamydia trachomatis*, Herpes simplex virus, Trichomonas vaginalis and *Neisseria gonorrhoeae*. *Human Path* 1990;**21**: 831–837.

16. Braley AE. Inclusion blenorrhea. A study of the pathologic changes in the conjunctiva and cervix. *Am J Ophthalmol* 1938;**21**:1203–1207.

17. Paavonen J, Vesterinen E, Meyer B, et al. Colposcopic and histologic findings of cervical chlaymdia infection. *Obstet Gynecol* 1990;**59**:712–771.

18. Seger F. The cytology of trachoma. *Am J Ophthalmol* 1951;**34**:1709–1713.

19. Greenwood SM, Moran TT. Chronic endometritis: Morphologic and clinical observations. *Obstet Gynecol* 1981;**58**:176–184.

20. Ingerslev HJ, Møller BR, Mardh P-A. *Chlamydia trachomatis* in acute and chronic endometritis. *Scand J Infect Dis* 1982;**32**(suppl):60–63.

21. Mardh P-A, Møller BR, Ingerselv HJ, Nussler E, Westrőm L, Wølner-Hanssen P. Endometritis caused by *Chlamydia trachomatis*. *Br J Vener Dis* 1981;**57**: 191–195.

22. Paavonen J, Aine R, Teisala K, Heinonnen PK, Punnonen R, Miettinen A, Gronroos P. Chlamydial endometritis. *J Clin Pathol* 1985;**38**:726–732.

23. Winkler B, Gallo L, Reumann W, Richart RM, Mitao M, Crum CP. Chlamydial

endometritis: A histological and immunohistochemical analysis. *Am J Surgical Path* 1984;**8**:771–778.

24. Winkler B, Crum CP. *Chlamydia trachomatis* infection of the female genital tract: Pathogenetic and clinicopathologic considerations, in Sommers SC, Feehner RE, Rosen PP (eds): *Pathol Annu.* E Norwalk, CT, Apple-Century-Crofts, 1987, 22 Pt. 1, pp. 193–223.

25. Crum CP, Egawa K, Fenoglio CM, Richart RM. Chronic endometritis: The role of immunohistochemistry in the detection of plasma cells. *Am J Obstet Gynecol* 1983;**147**(7):812–815.

26. Eduardo S, Tomioka ES, Anzai RY, Wu NK, Carvalho FM, Czeresnia CE, Petti DA, Peixoto S, de Souza AZ. Endometrial damage in acute salpingitis. *Sex Transm Dis* 1987;63–68.

27. Kiviat NB, Wølner-Hanssen P, Eschenbach DA, Wasserheit JN, Paavonen JA, Bell TA, Critchlow CW, Stamm WE, Moore DE, Holmes KK. Endometrial histophathology in patients with culture-proved upper genital tract infection and laparoscopically diagnosed acute salpingitis. *Am J Surg Pathol* 1990;**14**:167–175.

13
Behavioral Aspects of Pelvic Inflammatory Disease

Stuart N. Seidman and Sevgi Okten Aral

In many ways, pelvic inflammatory disease (PID) is a behavioral disease: its etiology involves the interaction of microorganisms with individual behavior, and its prevention and control require individual behavior change, including appropriate actions of clinicians and public health professionals. Our goal in this chapter is to examine the role of such behavior—of individuals, communities, and health-care providers—in the complex pathogenesis of PID and its sequelae. We will examine behavioral risk for PID in the context of the normal physiology and microbiology of the female genital tract, the different microorganisms that give rise to lower genital tract infection, and factors related to the ascendance of bacteria to the upper genital tract. In particular, we will focus on those behaviors that suggest interventions to reduce PID morbidity.

Overview

Most cases of PID begin in the lower genital tract. Cervical infection with sexually transmitted bacteria is directly linked to upper tract infection: *Neisseria gonorrhoeae* and/or *Chlamydia trachomatis* are isolated from the fallopian tubes in the majority of cases of PID in most series.[1,2,3] Furthermore, such pathogens may be partially responsible for some "endogenous" (i.e., non-STD) PID by damaging protective cervical mechanisms and allowing for the ascent of microorganisms.[4]

Alteration in the vaginal microenvironment, too, may be linked to the development of PID. The normal microbial flora of the vagina contains many species, dominated by lactobacilli.[5] Some studies suggest that vaginal lactobacilli, which produce hydrogen peroxide, in synergy with low pH, are protective against development of bacterial vaginosis (BV) and trichomoniasis, and perhaps gonorrhea and chlamydia.[6,7,8] Bacterial vaginosis is a condition in which the vaginal flora is altered to contain strictly anaerobic bacteria, in addition to the usual aerobic and facultative bacteria.[5,9] This may be an important initial step in the pathogenesis of some cases of PID: presence of BV has been associated with upper tract infection,[1,5] and the same spectrum of species can be isolated from the upper genital tract of some women with "endogenous" PID,[2,5] though such isolation is inconsistent.[3] One study of 642 women found adnexal tenderness to be significantly more common among women with evidence of BV than among those without it, even after controlling for the effects of other variables with multivariate analysis.[5] In addition, this condition may facilitate cervical infection with sexually transmitted pathogens.[4]

Behaviors that affect the initial stage of infection—either sexually transmitted lower genital tract infection or alteration of the vaginal microenvironment—will influence the later development of PID. Behaviors that have an impact on the microbial flora of the vagina include: having multiple sexual partners; vaginal douching; use of birth control methods, such as oral contraceptives (OCs) or spermicides; and use of lactobacilli-containing vaginal products.[7,8] Behaviors that increase an individual woman's risk of lower tract infection with gonorrhea or chlamydia include those that influence her partner's likelihood of infection (e.g., male behavior), those that increase her exposure to infected partners (e.g., having multiple partners), and/or those that enhance acquisition of infection given exposure (e.g., lack of barrier method use).

Importantly, most women who develop these preconditions to PID—acquisition of lower tract infection or disturbance of the normal vaginal flora—do not have typical symptoms (i.e., vaginal discharge). Thus, prevention of such lower tract conditions cannot rely only on treatment of symptomatic women. Provider behaviors such as screening, appropriate treatment, risk reduction counseling, and contact tracing are therefore important.

The second stage in the development of PID is the ascendance, or migration, of lower genital tract microorganisms to the upper genital tract.[10] After establishment of lower tract infection, ascendance of bacteria is blocked at the cervix and at the uterotubal junction. To breach these formidable barriers, some have suggested that microorganisms are transported on a vector, such as *T. vaginalis* or spermatozoa,[11] or are "sucked in" due to pressure changes during coitus.[12]

In each individual, the ascendance of bacteria, and thus risk for upper tract infection, is influenced by biological and behavioral factors. Individual suceptibility (e.g., immune response, cervical ectopy, and cervical mucus plug),[4] and characteristics of the specific pathogen are biological determinants of the likelihood of ascendance. The behavioral factors affecting ascendance are difficult to measure precisely. It is likely that behaviors associated with the progression of lower to upper tract infection include those that enhance ascendance itself, those that are markers of women who develop clinically diagnosed PID, and those provider and health-care behaviors that could prevent ascendance.

High coital frequency, vaginal douching, use or nonuse of certain contraceptives, and inadequate health-care behaviors are plausible mediators of enhanced ascendance of pathogens.[13-16] Tobacco smoking and other substance abuse, which are associated with upper tract infection, may play a role at this stage, or may be markers of other phenomena; little is known of the precise mechanisms mediating these associations.[14,16,17] Finally, health care is an important component of PID acquisition. Behaviors related to personal health care, such as symptom evaluation, health-care access, treatment compliance, and partner referral are associated with incidence of upper tract infection. Clinician and public health provider behaviors, such as appropriate screening, patient treatment, partner treatment, and counseling, are relevant for primary prevention (e.g., behavioral risk reduction), secondary prevention (e.g., screening), and possibly tertiary prevention (i.e., prevention of tubal sequelae).[18,19] Because undiagnosed PID is implicated in a growing proportion of cases of tubal infertility, tertiary prevention has become especially important.[15,18,19]

Sociodemographic factors are important markers of the incidence and course of sexually transmitted infection in general, and accordingly, they play an important role in reported PID incidence. Specifically, young age, minority race, low socioeconomic status (SES), and unmarried marital status are associated with diagnosed PID.[16] The implications of such sociodemographic factors for behavioral risk are substantial.

Behavioral Influences on the Stages of Pelvic Inflammatory Disease

The natural history of STD-associated PID highlights five progressive stages of infection for which behavioral risk may be determined: exposure to pathogenic bacteria, acquisition of infection upon exposure, development of symptomatic or asymptomatic lower tract disease, ascendance of bacteria with development of upper tract infection, and progression to severe or irreversible sequelae.[16,10] Risk behaviors associated with each of these stages may be amenable to intervention. Furthermore, provider behaviors that influence timely detection and treatment of genital tract infections can have a significant impact on PID morbidity.[19]

Exposure to Pathogenic Bacteria

Behaviors that mediate exposure to a sexually transmitted pathogen may be divided into those that increase the prevalence of urethral infection among the men who are potential partners of a particular group of women, the "partner pool"; and those that increase an individual woman's risk of choosing an infected partner. These factors are interrelated, in that women who are less discriminating in their partner choice often select partners from a group of men with a high prevalence of STD.[20]

Male Factors

The etiological agents of most urethritis in men can cause PID in women.[21] Thus, risk factors for male urethritis are directly linked to the occurrence of PID in female sex partners. For example, women whose male partners use condoms are at decreased risk for cervical gonorrhea and for hospitalization for PID compared to women whose partners do not use condoms.[22-26] Furthermore, in one large series etiological pathogens were isolated from the majority of the steady sex partners of women admitted for acute PID; such pathogens were asymptomatic in about three-fourths of the men from whom they were isolated.[27]

Little evidence exists from population-based samples describing risk factors for urethritis in men.[28,29] In addition to the presumed high-risk behaviors, sociodemographic factors have been associated with bacterial urethritis among some men. These include: age younger than 25 years,[21] African-American race,[28] and possibly low SES and urban residence;[28] such studies, however, are biased by their restriction to STD clinic populations. Available data indicate that these sociodemographic variables are likely markers for high-risk sexual and health-care-seeking behaviors, inadequate access to health care, and/or a high baseline prevalence of STD in the community, which, taken together, lead to a high incidence of all sexually transmitted infections. Risky behaviors include individual sexual and health-care-seeking behavior, those behaviors of sex partners, and relevant behavior of health-care providers.

Sexual behaviors that specifically increase the risk of male infection, and therefore of PID in their partners, are currently being defined. The consistent use of barrier methods in all sexual interactions protects a man from acquisition of urethritis.[30,31] Having multiple sex partners increases a man's risk for viral and bacterial STD,[32] though this is also a marker of a particularly "risky" partner recruitment strategy.[33,34] Similarly, cigarette smoking has been linked to urethritis, though this association may be spurious.[35] Finally, anything that increases their female partners' risk of acquiring, not being treated for, and/or transmitting gonococcal or chlamydial infection will increase the incidence of urethritis in a group of men. For example, the efficiency of chlamydial transmission may be greater to young females because of associated ectopy.[36] This would increase the prevalence of chlamydial cervicitis in young women, and increase the risk for urethritis among men who have sex with such women.

Health-care behaviors of men that are relevant to the potential spread of PID-associated bacteria are those that may hinder diagnosis and treatment of urethritis. These include: inadequate self-evaluation of symptoms, inappropriate treatment decisions (e.g., use of street antibiotics instead of STD clinic evaluation), noncompliance with treatment instructions (e.g., insufficient antimicrobial course), and lack of sex partner referral for STD evaluation.

Finally, screening and partner notification activities of the public health apparatus are related to STD prevalence, which indirectly affects each individual's risk of exposure to a pathogen. Asymptomatic infections, which may occur in one-fourth of men with chlamydial urethritis[36] and as many as two-thirds of women with chlamydial cervicitis,[37] are brought to treatment only through these activities. At the population level, when any of these factors prevents or delays the eradication of some proportion of pathogenic bacteria, more women will be exposed, and the incidence of PID will likely rise.

Female Factors

Among women, exposure to a partner infected with PID-causing bacteria depends primarily on partner recruitment strategy, and by extension, the particular pool of men from which they choose partners.[20,33] The propensity to choose an infected partner is related to the number of lifetime or recent partners, rate of acquisition of new partners, and age at first sexual intercourse.[38] These, in turn, are related to one another, and to a woman's partner recruitment strategy.[39] Each of these behavioral factors is associated with acquisition of lower tract infection with PID-associated bacteria,[40,41] and with PID itself.[13,14,16,22,23,42] At the population level, having multiple current partners is of further importance because in addition to increasing a woman's risk for acquisition of gonorrhea[43] and chlamydia,[37,40,44] this behavior leads to greater dissemination of these microorganisms in the population.

In addition to these sexual behaviors, the same sociodemographic risk markers (young age, black race, low SES, and urban residence) noted for male urethritis are associated with diagnosed lower tract infection in women.[45-48] This probably reflects exposure to a relatively circumscribed male partner pool with a high baseline prevalence of STD.

Acquisition of Lower Genital Tract Infection

All women do not develop endocervical infection following exposure to an infected sexual partner. The estimated male-to-female, transmission rate of gonorrhea is 43% to 100%; for chlamydia it is 9% to 40%.[49-52] Factors that mediate this process include: those related to the pathogenic bacteria, such as the size of the inoculum (which may be related to the stage of infection in the male), and the virulence of infecting pathogens;[16] those associated with host susceptibility, such as age, immune response to previous infection, and the changing nature of cervical mucus;[4] and behavioral/environmental factors. In addition, the ability to culture gonorrhea and chlamydia varies (e.g., with biological factors, or with external factors such as culture technique) leading to potentially biased interpretations of culture data.[4]

Clearly, the most important behavior that will prevent acquisition at this stage is the use of barrier contraceptive methods.[24,25,53] Consistent and correct condom use protects against acquisition of most STD[26,30,31,54,55] inconsistent use offers little protection.[30,54] Spermicides kill *N. gonorrhoeae* and *C. trachomatis*, and are associated with decreased risk for cervical infection with these organisms.[24,50,53,55-57] Diaphragm use is also associated with decreased risk for these cervical infections,[58-61] although this may reflect the protective effect of the spermicide with which it is typically used. Most, but not all, studies suggest that the combination of spermicide with latex condoms offers greater protection against acquisition of STD than either alone.[24,62] Recent data, however, have linked the use of spermicides to disturbance of the normal vaginal ecosystem, and to development of urinary tract infection.[63-65] Moreover, if BV is a risk factor for endogenous PID,[5] through this mechanism spermicide use may also increase risk for some upper tract infections. Further investigation is needed to clarify the net effects of spermicide use on risk of infection.

Use of contraceptives other than barrier methods have less impact on lower tract infection. The intrauterine device (IUD), tubal ligation, and withdrawal do not measurably alter STD risk. the influence of OCs on lower genital tract infections is uncertain, and may depend on age. *C. trachomatis* is more commonly cultured from the endocervix of women who use OCs than from those who do not use OCs.[4,37,66-68] However, whether the actual incidence of infection among these women is greater is not clear. Cervical changes induced by OCs, such as the increasesed amount of ectopic tissue, may lead to greater susceptibility to infection[69] or such changes may only increase the yield of chlamydia culture.[68] Oral contraceptive use may also be a marker for other factors associated with infection. However, a recent randomized prospective study that controlled for ectopy, demographics, and some behaviors found a 70% increased likelihood of gonorrheal or chlamydial infection among OC users compared to users of IUDs or tubal ligation.[68] This supports the conclusion that OCs promote acquisition of lower genital tract chlamydial infections.[51]

Sexual behaviors that are associated with acquisition of cervical infection, such as having multiple partners and a high rate of acquiring new partners,[33,38,41] may actually mediate exposure rather than acquisition, though it is difficult to establish at which stage of infection their influence is greatest. Greater coital frequency and earlier first intercourse, both associated with STD, and specifically with PID[13,14,16,22,23,70] may play a role in the development of lower tract infection given exposure(s) to an infected partner. Age is probably an important factor mediating acquisition, given its association with cervical ectopy and with behavior: in one study of adolescent women, only early first intercourse and years of sexual activity were associated with lower tract chlamydial infection.[66]

Timing of coitus in relation to menses,[71] female orgasm,[12] local genital hygiene after coitus,[26] vaginal douching,[72,73] use of prophylactic antibiotics,[26] cigarette smoking,[14,17,74] and substance abuse[72] have each been proposed as possible mediators of lower and upper tract infection. Firm evidence of their causal association with acquisition of cervical infection, however, is lacking. For now, they remain issues for further research.

Behavioral factors that facilitate the development of BV, because of the potential relationship to endogenous PID, deserve attention here as modifiable risk factors for lower tract "disease." The vaginal flora varies with the menstrual cycle, sexual intercourse, pregnancy, contraceptive use, and age.[5,8,75] Lactobacillus species that produce hydrogen peroxide, in synergy with low pH, act as functional barriers against disturbance of the normal vaginal ecosystem.[6-8] One longitudinal study suggests that women with such lactobacillia are one-seventh as likely to develop BV and trichomoniasis, compared to women with nonperoxide-producing lactobacilli, even after adjustment for demographic and behavioral factors.[8] These lactobacilli may also be protective against gonorrheal and chlamydial infections.[8] The impact of behaviors that disturb this ecosystem, such as vaginal douching, having multiple partners, spermicide use, and IUD use are poorly understood. Further research is needed to better define the link between behavior and the vaginal microenvironment, and this environment and PID.

Potential Treatment of Lower Genital Tract Infection

Most cases of cervicitis are asymptomatic.[9,51] At the cervical stage of infection, prompt diagnosis, treatment, and partner treatment are critical: upper tract infection may be prevented, and further transmission of pathogenic bacteria may be stopped. In the population, then, behaviors that delay eradication of pathogenic bacteria (from the individual and the community) will lead to an increase in PID-associated morbidity. These include inadequate self-evaluation of symptoms, inappropriate or delayed treatment seeking, having sex after symptoms appear, noncompliance with treatment instructions, and/or lack of sex partner referral for STD evaluation.[22,76] Sexually transmitted disease prevalence will remain high among groups of men and women who have less access to health care (e.g., from lower SES); who tend to delay treatment seeking (e.g., adolescents); and/or who are counseled in a culturally inappropriate way (e.g., in a language that is poorly understood).

Most cases of cervicitis are diagnosed through screening and partner notification; most upper tract infections, and most female-to-male transmission occur in the context of asymptomatic cervical infections (i.e., those without self-recognized purulent discharge). Health-care-provider behaviors affecting treatment of such cervical infections are, thus, especially important for preventing ascendance of pathogens to the upper genital tract, and for halting further transmission.[15] These behaviors include screening of high-risk populations, appropriate sign/symptom evaluation, appropriate treatment, partner notification, and risk reduction counseling.

Ascendance to Upper Genital Tract/Development of PID

Untreated, 10% to 50% of cervical infections with gonorrhea or chlamydia will lead to PID.[50,51] Factors that are associated with migration of lower tract pathogens to the upper genital tract are difficult to determine because the lower tract infections that do come to medical attention are treated, and most lower and upper tract infections are asymptomatic or atypical. Thus, it is virtually impossible to study the natural course of untreated genital tract infection. Nonetheless, risk factors for PID that are distinct from risk factors for cervicitis are most likely related to the ascendance of pathogens. Such factors are just beginning to be elucidated with study designs comparing patients diagnosed with PID to those with cervicitis only.[71]

Normally, the upper genital tract is sterile. Endometrial colonization, however, appears to be relatively common,[4] and it is likely that a considerable "microbial traffic" occurs between the endocervix, the endometrium, and the fallopian tubes.[1,4,10,77–80] The cervix is thought to be a functional barrier to the ascent of microorganisms, protecting upper tract sterility. This cervical barrier is mechanical, biochemical, and immunological.[2,4] It is attributable to the cervical mucus plug and to components of cervical secretions, both of which vary under the influence of hormones.[4,81] The mechanisms of this stage of infection are poorly elucidated. It may be that propulsion of bacteria into the fallopian tubes is the initiating event in upper tract disease. Any factor that reduces the protective value of the cervical barrier or enhances microbial ascendance is assumed to increase the likelihood of upper tract infection.

The use of mechanical and chemical barriers, noted above as protective against lower tract infections, is also associated with a lower risk of PID relative to nonusers of any method; the diaphragm offers the greatest protection, and spermicide alone the least ($RR = 0.3–0.9$).[22,24,25,53,55,70] Use of barrier methods is also associated with lower rates of tubal infertility,[82,83] and tubal pregnancy.[84] It is unclear, however, whether this is due only to a lowered incidence of sexually transmitted cervicitis, or to some other mechanism that protects from upper tract infection after acquisition of lower tract infection, and/or reduces sequelae.[15] In addition, recent concerns about the effect of spermicide use on the vaginal flora, and implications for PID acquisition have not been resolved.[6–8]

Pelvic inflammatory disease risk is greatest for women with multiple lifetime partners,[13,14,22,23] multiple current partners,[22,42] and early first sexual intercourse.[13,70,72,85] Furthermore, it is known to be more common among young, unmarried, and black women.[13,42,86] Whether these associations are mediated only by the already established association with lower tract infection, or by some other mechanism occurring later in the progression to upper tract infection, is undetermined.

In contrast, vaginal douching is not associated with a greater risk for lower tract infection (and may even be somewhat protective),[16] but does increase risk for acute PID.[16,72,73] Women with acute PID are more likely to have a history of douching than are women without PID.[13,72,73,87] In one case-control study in which multivariate analysis was used to adjust for confounding, douching during the past 2 months was associated with a relative risk of 1.7 (95% $CI = 1.0–2.8$) for PID.[72] No particular douching method or fluid was more consistently associated with PID, but greater frequency of douching increased PID risk.[72]

A greater frequency of intercourse, too, is associated with increased PID risk,[14,22,23,42,70] especially among presumably monogamous women.[42,88] As a risk factor for acute, hospitalized PID in one case-control study, intercourse more than five times per week gave a relative risk of 1.7 (95% $CI = 1.2–2.4$) for all women, and 3.2 (95% $CI = 1.7–5.7$) for monogamous women (relative to similar women who had intercourse ≤5 times per week).[42] Although douching and coital frequency are possibly only markers for other factors, these behaviors offer a plausible mechanism for the ascendance of pathogenic bacteria to the upper tract. Each could alter the vaginal microenvironment in ways conducive to the growth of pathogenic organisms, or facilitate ascendance of such organisms. Appropriate studies to test these hypotheses have not been done, or are inconclusive.

Timing of behavioral exposure is a potentially important aspect of upper genital tract infection, especially with respect to menses, or uterine propulsive activity. Onset of symptomatic upper tract infection with chlamydia and/or gonorrhea is more common within 7 days of the onset of menses than at other times in the cycle[4,15,89,90]; the reverse is true of "endogenous" PID.[15,16,89] After ovulation (under the influence of progesterone produced by the corpus luteum), cervical mucus becomes more viscous, and acts as a plug to seal off the uterine cavity.[4] During menses, after expulsion of the plug, bacteria may gain access to the uterus, or be propelled into the fallopian tubes by uterine contractions during sloughing.[2,4] Uterine contractions are also known to occur in association with orgasm[91] and IUD use, and are decreased by progesterone administration.[92] The behavioral implications of these potential high-risk time periods for ascendance of pathogens have not been fully explored. In one study of 500 infertile patients, coitus during menses was not associated with PID or with tubal infertility.[93] However, a case-control study comparing 135 women with PID to 740 randomly selected controls from and STD clinic population revealed that coitus during menses and prolonged bleeding during menses increased risk for gonococcal and endogenous PID, but not gonococcal cervicitis or any chlamydial genital tract infection.[71]

Overall, OC use is associated with a lower risk of symptomatic, clinically overt PID,[16,22,25,67,90,94–102] and no increase or a decrease in tubal infertility.[82,83] Possible mechanisms of estrogen or progesterone influence may be through directly affecting the growth of microorganisms[4]; through decreased menstrual blood loss (providing a more hostile environment for bacterial proliferation)[16]; through thickened cervical mucus (forming a less penetrable barrier)[16]; through greater growth of target epithelial cells and the development of cervical ectopy[4]; or through altering the immune response to chlamydial infection.[16] Since detection of cervical chlamydia is greater from women using OCs[37,66,69,103–105] and a large proportion of PID is atypical and remains undetected,[45,106] the net effect of OC use on chlamydial PID remains unclear.[16,51,67,107,108] Available data suggest a lowered risk for development[101,109] and less severe clinical course of chlamydial PID,[2,22,51,95,101] and no effect on gonococcal PID.[22]

Cigarette smoking and substance abuse have each been linked specifically to PID, though the causal mechanisms are undetermined.[15] Two studies have found that cigarette smoking doubles the PID risk.[14,17,110] Alcohol and cocaine use have been associated with gonorrhea and with PID.[72,111] It is difficult, however, to determine whether these factors are markers for other primary mechanisms, or are themselves associated with some unknown biological risk.

Although the mechanism of STD-associated bacterial ascendance is poorly elucidated, other upper tract infections are clearly the result of direct introduction of pathogens during medical procedures, so called "iatrogenic ascendance." These include cases of PID that follow uterine instrumentation, up to 12% of PID cases in one series.[106] Insertion of an IUD, in particular, increases the risk of PID by 1.5–2.6 times, especially during the first few months after insertion, and among women with BV.[2,16,88,94] Organisms from the vagina and/or cervix are probably directly introduced to the uterus during insertion.[26] However, the increased risk is transient,[23] apparently associated mostly with use of the Dalkon Shield™,[109] (though this is disputed by some),[112] minimal among women at low risk of acquiring STD,[23] and reduced by the prophylactic use of doxycycline at the time of IUD insertion.[16] Thus, for women who are at low risk for STD acquisition, insertion of currently available IUDs with prophylactic doxycycline administration and careful follow-up may not increase PID risk at all.[26,113,114,115]

Progression to Tubal Damage

The most serious complication of PID is tubal damage, and consequent impairment of fertility, ectopic pregnancy, and/or chronic pelvic pain. Preventing progression of upper genital tract infection to tubal dysfunction and/or obstruction is usually impossible, even with the substantial impact of antibiotics on symptoms of acute infection.[71] Thus, once tubal damage has begun, it is unclear if intervention influences the risk of adverse sequelae. This is difficult to establish definitively, because most cases of presumptive salpingitis that have been retrospectively associated with such sequelae (i.e., through serological tests for past chlamydial infection) were subclinical.[51]

Factors that are associated with a greater incidence of tubal infertility and ectopic pregnancy after clinically apparent PID include age older than 25 years, number and severity of infections,[106,108,116] and perhaps cigarette smoking,[117,118] contraceptive choice, and timeliness of institution of appropriate antimicrobial therapy.[16,19] As expected, factors that reduce the incidence of PID (such as use of barrier methods) are also associated with lowered rates of tubal infertility,[82] and ectopic pregnancy.[84]

Behaviors relevant to the development of sequelae after PID include OC use, vaginal douching, and health-care/provider behaviors that detect asymptomatic disease. Oral contraceptive use is associated with no increase, and perhaps a decrease in tubal infertility, although this is somewhat controversial.[16,22,26,82,119] Ectopic pregnancy is relatively rare among women who use OCs (and other forms of contraception) consistently, although failure of tubal sterilization is associated with an increased risk for an ectopic pregnancy.[119] In a case-control study of 306 patients with ectopic pregnancies compared to 266 with intrauterine pregnancies, serological evidence of past chlamydial exposure, and vaginal douching were independently associated with increased risk for ectopic pregnancy ($OR = 3.0$ and 2.1, respectively).[120] The association of vaginal douching with an increased rate of tubal pregnancy has been noted in other studies,[121,122] but it is unclear whether it specifically increases risk for this sequelae.[16] Similarly, cigarette smoking is associated with an increased risk of ectopic pregnancy[117] and infertility,[118] but whether smoking increases risk of sequelae after acute PID has not been addressed.[16]

Perhaps most important in the prevention of adverse sequelae is the recognition of the existence and implications of asymptomatic upper tract disease. In addition to the clinically apparent cases of PID affecting over a million women in the United States each year, evidence of an epidemic of "silent PID" is growing.[51,106] A large proportion of cases of chlamydial salpingitis, especially, may produce symptoms so minimal that they are not brought to medical attention, or are misdiagnosed. There is a higher prevalence of antichlamydial antibodies among women with infertility due to tubal disease compared to those with infertility due to other causes,[51,120,123,124] and among women with ectopic pregnancies.[51,103,125] Risk factors for silent PID are difficult to establish, much less intervene with.[83] Thus, to have an appreciable impact on PID-related complications, pathogenic organisms will need to be eradicated before they reach the fallopian tubes; intervention cannot wait for the development of symptoms. This challenges the behavior of the patient, the health-care provider, and the public health apparatus.

Sociodemographic Risk Factors for PID

An important component of behavioral intervention is targeting specific women at high risk for development of PID because of specific high-risk behaviors. Some high-risk behaviors and high-risk partners are more common among certain sociodemographic groups of women, and the relative importance of different behavioral risk factors for PID varies among such groups. In particular, marital status, age, race, and SES describe groups of women whose sexual behavior and partner pools are somewhat distinct.[126] In many studies. having multiple partners has been shown to increase the risk for PID[13,14,16,45,127]; reducing the number of partners is a major goal of behavioral intervention for women among whom having multiple current partners is most prevalent, such as younger, never married white women, and older, formerly married black women.[39,128,129] Among women who have only one partner, other factors, such as vaginal douching, frequency of intercourse, and partner behavior may be more appropriate for intervention.

An accurate description of the epidemiology of PID is limited by the inadequacy of population-based surveillance of upper tract infection. Incidence data for PID are scant; the best population-based samples are women hospitalized for PID,[86] and representative surveys of reproductive-age American women.[13] These samples are not representative of all women with upper genital tract infections: women hospitalized with acute PID account for an estimated one-fourth (and most severe) of all cases of acute PID, and "endogenous" PID is likely overrepresented[130]; surveys depend on self-report, and are thus subject to recall bias. Nonetheless, from them some important inferences may be made about PID incidence, and perhaps etiology.

The incidence of gonorrheal and chlamydial lower and upper tract infections are highest among young women[2,15,45,72,108,127]; the rate of severe PID sequelae, however, is the lowest among young women.[2,16] Sexually experienced teenagers are three times more likely to be diagnosed with PID than are those in their late 20s.[16] Biology and behavior play a role in these phenomena. Younger women are more likely to have more than one current sex partner,[39] and to have had an early age at first sexual intercourse[131]; these are both associated with increased PID risk.[13,45,85,127] Cervical ectopy occurs more commonly among younger women; this and other age-related changes in endocervical defense mechanisms or mucus may determine the fate of lower genital tract infections.[4,16,45] In addition, adolescents tend to delay seeking treatment once symptoms arise.[132] Thus, the pathogenesis of PID, and presumably the relative influence of different behavioral factors, is probably different among younger women compared to older women.

Similarly, SES and race distinguish women with distinct risks for PID acquisition. These markers are difficult to untangle because they are associated with one another, and because most American studies of PID have not adequately distinguished SES from race. Still, it is well established that both low SES and minority race are associated with elevated risk for PID.[16] Various measures of low SES have been associated with an increased risk of PID.[13,14,16,22,72] Young black women, who have the highest incidence of PID,[16,45,108,127] are at greatly elevated risk of lower tract infection per sexual encounter due to the high prevalence of infection in their partner pool.[16] In a sample of 8,450 American women surveyed in 1988, having multiple lifetime sex partners increased black women's risk for PID disproportionately compared to white women.[13] Multivariate analysis of the same database revealed unmarried marital status, vaginal douching, and early age at first intercourse to be associated with a history of PID among white women but not among black women.[13] Thus, behavioral risk for PID among black women may be especially influenced by the behavior of their partners.[133]

Unmarried marital status is a risk factor for acute PID,[16] although this may be true only for white women.[13] The 1979–1988 average annual number of hospital admissions for acute PID, however, was almost equal among married women (68,750) to that among unmarried women (75,490); the incidence rate, too, was substantial among married women (2.37 per 1,000 compared to 3.84 per 1,000 among unmarried women).[86] In a study for which age adjustment was made, the rate of acute, hospitalized PID was not significantly lower among married compared to unmarried women.[42] Because having multiple partners is rare among married women,[39,129] most of the PID due to sexually transmitted pathogens among these women is probably accounted for by the risky behavior of their husbands (i.e., having other female partners without using barrier methods). It is also possible that a greater proportion of endogenous PID occurs among married women than among unmarried women.

Among women with only one current sex partner, a high frequency of intercourse and vaginal douching may be particularly important risk factors for PID. From a multicenter, hospital-based, case-control study of PID conducted from 1976 to 1978, in a subset of presumably monogamous women (i.e., currently married, reporting one sexual partner in the preceding 6 months), those who reported having sex six or more times a week were more likely to have PID than similar women who had sex less frequently ($OR = 3.2$, 95% $CI = 1.7$–5.7).[42] In a study of IUD use, the risk for PID among women who had only one sexual partner was more correlated with frequency of intercourse than with IUD use.[88] Vaginal douching is associated with PID most strongly among women with 10 or fewer lifetime sexual partners ($OR = 3.5$, 95% $CI = 1.9$–6.4), and less so among those with more than 10 lifetime partners.[72] Although these behaviors are probably also important among women at higher risk for STD, the strength of the association of STD with PID masks that relationship.

Provider Behavior

Relevant clinician and public health system influences noted above need to be delineated specifically for use in intervention strategies. It is clear that at each stage in the pathogenesis of upper tract infection, appropriate intervention can abort the progression of disease, and effectively prevent sequelae. Furthermore, early diagnosis and treatment not only protects the reproductive health of the infected individual, but reduces further transmission of pathogenic bacteria.

The provider of STD services, in addition to the traditional responsibility for treatment of disease, must take an active role in prevention of STD, especially in high-risk populations. Specifically, the Centers for Disease Control (CDC) has recommended five components of effective provider behavior aimed at reducing PID morbidity[15]: (1) maintain a current knowledge base about STD/PID prevention and control; (2) provide STD preventive services, especially screening of high-risk groups, and presumptive (and epidemiologic) treatment of high-risk patients; (3) treat STD appropriately; (4) ensure treatment of infected partners; and (5) provide risk-reduction counseling.

The basis for timely and appropriate implementation of these priorities depends on knowledge of the individual patient's risk for disease. For example, in a study of cervicitis in 680 Indonesian women, using five factors to develop a risk profile, it was possible to distinguish high-risk women (with a 17% prevalence of culture-proven cervicitis) from low-risk women (with less than 1% prevalence of cervicitis).[134] Such a risk assessment will impact the clinician's diagnostic and treatment decisions, as well as primary prevention activities.

Risk-reduction counseling, in particular, focuses on behaviors that contribute to an individual's STD risk. Its aim is to promote safer sexual behavior practices by informing the high-risk patient about behaviors that are especially risky, and those that reduce risk.[15] The clinician is in a unique position to encourage realistic, healthy behavior change, and this opportunity for prevention should not be missed.

Prevention of PID

As described above, behaviors are important influences on the course of upper genital tract infection, and effective prevention is possible through behavioral intervention. In fact, PID, although caused by the action of pathogenic bacteria in the upper genital tract, is in large part a behavioral disease: it is inextricably tied to the behaviors of men and women that increase transmission of these pathogens; of women, in particular, which increase their own risk for acquisition of lower genital tract infection; and of the providers of clinical and preventive services responsible for STD treatment and prevention.

On the basis of what is known about behavioral influences on the stages of lower and upper genital tract infection, guidelines for primary, secondary, and tertiary prevention of PID have been developed with respect to communities, individuals, and health-care providers.[15,18] Full discussion of these strategies is beyond the scope of this chapter, but they have been lucidly described in recent comprehensive reviews,[16,26,135] and a CDC-issued report.[15] In general, community approaches involve maintaining health promotion and education messages, training health-care providers in STD prevention, and providing for appropriate screening, clinical services, and partner notification activities.[15]

Some behaviors can be specifically linked to a decrease in an individual's risk for developing PID: compliance with treatment for STD, limiting the number of sex partners, and using barrier contraceptive methods.[15] Although proper evaluation studies have not been done, most authorities would, in addition, recommend maintenance of healthy sexual behaviors, such as avoidance of sex with an infected person, with casual partners, or when STD symptoms in oneself appear, and postponing the initiation of first intercourse until at least 2 to 3 years following menarche; adopting appropriate health-care-seeking behaviors, such as seeking care promptly if one may be at risk for having acquired an STD, getting screened regularly if not in a mutually monogamous relationship, complying with STD treatment instructions, and ensuring treatment of infected partners.[15]

Conclusion

Individual and community behaviors are important factors affecting the acquisition and course of genital tract infections. Given the burden of unrecognized infection in the population, maximally effective intervention strategies for PID will have to focus on prevention of cervical infection. Behavioral factors important for primary prevention of cervical infection are those that affect the prevalence of untreated urethritis among men (e.g., male health-seeking), and those that affect a woman's exposure to and acquisition of pathogens from such men (e.g., number of partners, condom use).

Once cervical infection is established, behavioral factors that are important mediators of ascendance to the upper genital tract and development of sequelae are poorly characterized. Further research to describe the role of potential mediators of ascendance, such as vaginal douching, coital frequency, timing of intercourse, and contraceptive choice, is crucial for the development of secondary prevention strategies. Overall, it is clear that reduction of PID and its sequelae through behavior change is an attainable public health objective.

Acknowledgments

We thank Ward Cates, Jr, MD, MPH, Stuart Berman, MD, Bob Johnson, MD, and Polly Marchbanks, PhD for their critical reviews and insightful comments.

References

1. Paavonen J, Teisala K, Heinonnen PK, et al. Microbiological and histological findings in acute pelvic inflammatory disease. *Br J Obstet Gynecol* 1987; **94**:454.
2. Weström L, Mardh P-A. Acute pelvic inflammatory disease, in Holmes KK, Mardh P-A, Sparling PF, Wiesner PJ (eds): *Sexually Transmitted Diseases*, 2nd ed. New York, McGraw-Hill International Book Co., 1990, pp 593–613.
3. Faro S, Martens M, Maccato M, Hammill H, Pearlman M. Vaginal flora and pelvic inflammatory disease. *Am J Obstet Gynecol* 1993;**169**:470–474.
4. Rice PA, Schachter J. Pathogenesis of pelvic inflammatory disease: What are the questions? *JAMA* 1991;**266**:2587–2593.
5. Spiegel CA. Bacterial vaginosis. *Clin Microbiol Rev* 1991;**4**:485–502.
6. Klebanoff SJ, Hillier SL, Eschenbach DA, Waltersdorph AM. Control of the microbial flora of the vagina by H_2O_2-generating lactobacilli. *J Infect Dis* 1991;**164**:94–100.
7. Hughes VL, Hillier SL. Microbiologic characteristics of lactobacillus products used for colonization of the vagina. *Obstet Gynecol* 1990;**75**:244–248.
8. Hillier S. The vagina as an ecosystem. *Presented at the International Society of STD Research 9th International Meeting*. Banff, Alberta, Canada, Oct. 6–9, 1991.
9. Holmes KK. Lower genital tract infections in women: Cystitis, urethritis, vulvovaginitis, and cervicitis, in Holmes KK, Mardh P-A, Sparling PF, Wiesner PJ (eds): *Sexually Transmitted Diseases*, 2nd ed. New York, McGraw-Hill International Book Co., 1990, pp 527–545.
10. Weström L, Wølner-Hanssen P. Pathogenesis of pelvic inflammatory disease. *Genitourin Med* 1993;**69**:9–17.
11. Keith LG, Berger GS, Edelman DA, et al. On the causation of pelvic inflammatory disease. *Am J Obstet Gynecol* 1984;**149**:215–223.
12. Fox CH, Wolff HS, Baker JA. Measurement of intravaginal and intrauterine pressures during human coitus by radio-telemetry. *J Reprod Fertil* 1970; **22**:243–251.
13. Aral SO, Mosher WD, Cates W Jr. Self reported pelvic inflammatory disease in the U.S., 1988. *JAMA* 1991;**266**:2570–2573.
14. Marchbanks PA, Lee NC, Peterson HB. Cigarette smoking as a risk factor for pelvic inflammatory disease. *Am J Obstet Gynecol* 1990;**162**:639–644.
15. Centers for Disease Control. Pelvic inflammatory disease: Guidelines for prevention and management. *MMWR* 1991;**40**:1–25.
16. Washington AE, Aral SO, Wølner-Hanssen P, Grimes DA, Holmes KK. Assessing risk for pelvic inflammatory disease and its sequelae. *JAMA* 1991;**266**:2581–2586.
17. Scholes D, Daling JR, Stergachis A. Current cigarette smoking and risk of acute pelvic inflammatory disease. *Am J Public Health* 1992;**82**:1352–1355.
18. Rolfs RT. "Think PID" New directions in prevention and management of PID. *Sex Transm Dis* 1991;**18**:131–132.
19. Hillis SD, Joesoef R, Marchbank PA, Wasserheit JN, Cates W Jr. Delayed care of pelvic inflammatory disease as a risk factor for impaired fertility. *Am J Obstet Gynecol* 1993;**168**:1503–1509.

20. Aral SO, Soskolne V, Joesoef RM, O'Reilly KR. Sex partner selection as risk factor for STD: Clustering of risky modes. *Sex Transm Dis* 1991;**18**: 10–17.

21. Rein MF. Urethritis, in Mandell GL, Douglas RG, Bennett JE (eds): *Principles and Practice of Infectious Disease*, 3rd ed. New York, Churchill Livingstone, Inc., 1990, pp 942–952.

22. Wølner-Hanssen P, Eschenbach DA, Paavonen J, et al. Decreased risk of symptomatic chlamydial pelvic inflammatory disease associated with oral contraceptive use. *JAMA* 1990;**263**:54–59.

23. Lee NC, Rubin GL, Borucki R. The intrauterine device and pelvic inflammatory disease revisited: New results from the Women's Health Study. *Obstet Gynecol* 1988;**72**:1–6.

24. Austin H, Louv WC, Alexander WJ. A case-control study of spermicides and gonorrhea. *JAMA* 1984;**251**:2822–2824.

25. Kelaghan J, Rubin GL, Ory HW, et al. Barrier-method contraceptives and pelvic inflammatory disease. *JAMA* 1982;**248**:184–187.

26. Washington AE, Cates W Jr, Wasserheit JN. Preventing pelvic inflammatory disease. *JAMA* 1991;**266**:2574–2580.

27. Kamwendo F, Johansson E, Moi H, Forslin L, Danielsson D. Gonorrhea, genital chlamydial infection, and nonspecific urethritis in male partners of women hospitalized and treated for acute pelvic inflammatory disease. *Sex Transm Dis* 1993;**20**:143–146.

28. Stamm WE, Koutsky LA, Benedetti JK, et al. *Chlamydia trachomatis* urethral infections in men. *Ann Int Med* 1984;**100**:47–51.

29. Morton WE, Horton HB, Baker HW. Effects of socioeconomic status on incidences of three sexually transmitted diseases. *Sex Transm Dis* 1979;**6**: 206–210.

30. Centers for Disease Control. Condoms for prevention of sexually transmitted diseases. *MMWR* 1988;**37**:133–137.

31. Darrow WW. Condom use and use-effectiveness in high-risk populations. *Sex Transm Dis* 1989;**16**:157–160.

32. Quinn RW, O'Reilly KR, Khaw M. Gonococcal infections in women attending the venereal disease clinic of the Nashville Davidson County Metropolitan Health Department, 1984. *South Med J* 1988;**81**:851–854.

33. Dan B. Sex and the singles' whirl: The quantum dynamics of Hepatitis B. *JAMA* 1986;**256**:1344.

34. Alter MJ, Ahtone J, Weisfuse I, Starko K, Vacalis TD, Maynard JE. Hepatitis B virus transmission between heterosexuals. *JAMA* 1986;**256**:1307–1310.

35. Pessione F, Dolivo M, Casin I, et al. Sexual behavior and smoking: Risk factor for urethritis in men. *Sex Transm Dis* 1988;**15**:119–122.

36. Stamm WE, Cole B. Asymptomatic *Chlamydia trachomatis* urethritis in men. *Sex Transm Dis* 1986;**13**:163–165.

37. Schachter J, Stoner E, Moncada J. Screening for chlaymdia infections in women attending family planning clinics. *West J Med* 1983;**138**:375–379.

38. Greenberg JB, Magder L, Aral SO. Age at first coitus: A marker for risky sexual behavior in women. *Sex Transm Dis* 1992;**19**:331–334.

39. Seidman SN, Mosher WD, Aral SO. Women with multiple sexual partners: USA, 1988. *Am J Pub Health* 1992;**82**:1388–1394.

40. Handsfield HH, Jasman LL, Roberts PL, Hanson VW, Kothenbeutal RL, Stamm WE. Criteria for selective screening for *Chlamydia trachomatis* in women attending family planning clinics. *JAMA* 1986;**255**:1730–1734.
41. D'Costa LJ, Plummer FA, Bowner I, et al. Prostitutes are a major reservoir of sexually transmitted diseases in Nairobi, Kenya. *Sex Transm Dis* 1985;**12**: 64–67.
42. Lee NC, Rubin GL, Grimes DA. Measures of sexual behavior and the risk of pelvic inflammatory disease. *Obstet Gynecol* 1991;**77**:425–430.
43. Pederson AHB, Bonin P. Screening females for asymptomatic gonorrhea infection. *Northwest J Med* 1971;**70**:255–261.
44. Johnson BA, Poses RM, Fortner CA, Meier FA, Dalton HP. Derivation and validation of a clinical diagnostic model for chlamydial cervical infection in university women. *JAMA* 1990;**264**:3161–3170.
45. Cates W Jr, Rolfs RT Jr, Aral SO. Sexually transmitted diseases, pelvic inflammatory disease, and infertility: An epidemiologic update. *Epidemiol Rev* 1990;**12**:199–220.
46. Aral SO, Holmes KK. Sexually transmitted diseases in the AIDS era. *Sci Am* 1991;**264**:62–69.
47. Aral SO, Holmes KK. Descriptive epidemiology of sexual behavior and sexually transmitted diseases, in Holmes KK, Mardh, P-A, Sparling PF, et al. (eds): *Sexually Transmitted Diseases*, 2nd ed. New York: McGraw-Hill 1990: 19–36.
48. Handsfield HH, Rice RJ, Roberts MC, Holmes KK. Localized outbreak of penicillinase-producing *Neisseria gonorrhoeae. JAMA* 1989;**261**: 2357–2361.
49. McCutchan JA. Epidemiology of venereal urethritis: Comparison of Gonorrhea and nongonococcal urethritis. *Rev Infect Dis* 1984;**6**:669.
50. Platt R, Rice PA, McCormack WM. Risk of acquiring gonorrhea and prevalence of abnormal adnexal findings among women recently exposed to gonorrhea. *JAMA* 1983;**250**:3205.
51. Cates W, Wasserheit JN. Genital chlamydial infections: Epidemiology and reproductive sequelae. *Am J Obstet Gynecol* 1991;**164**:1771–1781.
52. Katz BP, Caine VA, Jones RB. Estimation of transmission probabilities for chlamydial infection, in Bowie WR, Caldwell HD, Jones RB, et al. (eds): *Chlamydial Infections*. Cambridge, Cambridge University Press, 1990, pp 567–570.
53. Grimes DA, Cates W. Family planning and sexually transmitted diseases, in Holmes KK, Mardh P-A, Sparling PF, et al. (eds): *Sexually Transmitted Diseases*, 2nd ed. New York, McGraw-Hill, 1990, pp 1087–1094.
54. Instructions for condom use. Population Reports Series L:6,XIV:3,Pl-274. Baltimore, MD, The Johns Hopkins University, 1986.
55. Stone KR, Grimes DA, Magder LS. Personal protection against sexually transmitted diseases. *Am J Obstet Gynecol* 1986;**155**:180–188.
56. Louv WC, Austin H, Alexander WJ, Stagno S, Cheeks J. A clinical trial of nonoxynol-9 for preventing gonococcal and chlamydial infections. *J Infect Dis* 1988;**158**:518–523.
57. Rosenberg MJ, Rojanapithayakorn W, Feldblum PJ, Higgins JE. Effect of the contraceptive sponge on chlamydial infection, gonorrhea, and candidiasis: A comparative clinical trial. *JAMA* 1987:2308–2312.

58. Austin H, Louv WC, Alexander WJ. A case-control study of spermicides and gonorrhea. *JAMA* 1984;**251**:2822.
59. Quinn RW, O'Reilly KR. Contraceptive practices of women attending the sexually transmitted disease clinic in Nashville, Tennessee. *Sex Transm Dis* 1985;**12**:29.
60. Bradbeer CS, This RN, Tan T, Thirumoorthy T. Prophylaxis against infection in Singaporean prostitutes. *Genitourin Med* 1988;**64**:52–53.
61. Magder LS, Harrison HR, Ehret JM, Anderson TS, Judson FN. Factors related to genital chlamydia trachomatis and its diagnosis by culture in a sexually transmitted disease clinic. *Am J Epidemiol* 1988;**128**:298–308.
62. Judson FN, Ehret JM, Bolin GF, Levin MJ, Rietmeijer CAM. Unpublished data, 1992.
63. Hooton TM, Hillier S, Johnson C, Roberts PL, Stamm WE. Escherichia coli bacteriuria and contraceptive method. *JAMA* 1991;**265**:64–69.
64. Hooton TM, Fihn SD, Johnson C, Roberts PL, Stamm WE. Association between bacterial vaginosis and acute cystitis in women using diaphragms. *Arch Intern Med* 1989;**149**:1932–1936.
65. Hillier S, Hooton TM, Personal communication.
66. Shafer M-A, Beck A, Blain B, Dole P, Irwin CE Jr, Sweet R, Schachter J. *Chlamydia trachomatis*: Important relationships to race, contraception, lower genital tract infection, and Papanicolaou smear. *J Pediatr* 1984;**104**: 141–146.
67. Washington AE, Gove GF, Schachter J, Sweet RL. Oral contraceptives, *Chlamydia trachomatis* infection, and pelvic inflammatory disease: A word of caution about protection. *JAMA* 1985;**253**:2246–2250.
68. Louv WC, Austin H, Perlman J, Alexander WJ. Oral contraceptive use and the risk of chlamydial and gonococcal infections. *Am J Obstet Gynecol* 1989;**160**:396.
69. Ripa KT, Svensson L, Mardh P-A, et al. *Chlamydia trachomatis* cervicitis in gynecologic outpatients. *Obstet Gynecol* 1978;**52**:698–702.
70. Lidegaard D, Helm P. Pelvic inflammatory disease: The influence of contraceptive, sexual, and social life events. *Contraception* 1990;**41**:475–483.
71. Eschenbach D, Stevens C, Critchlow C, Holmes KK. Epidemiology of acute PID. *Presented at the International Society of STD Research 9th International Meeting.* Banff, Alberta, Canada, Oct. 6–9, 1991.
72. Wølner-Hanssen P, Eschenbach DA, Paavonen J, et al. Association between vaginal douching and acute pelvic inflammatory disease. *JAMA* 1990;**263**:1936–1941.
73. Scholes D, Daling JR, Stergachis A, Weiss NS, Wang SP, Grayston JT. Vaginal douching as a risk factor for acute pelvic inflammatory disease. *Obstet Gynecol* 1993;**81**:601–606.
74. Daling JR, Sherman KJ, Weisss NS. Risk factors for condyloma acuminatum in women. *Sex Transm Dis* 1986;**13**:16–18.
75. Kivijarvi A, Jarvinen H, Gronroos M. Microbiology of vaginitis associated with the intrauterine contraceptive device. *Br J Obstet Gynecol* 1984;91: 917–923.
76. Platt R, Rice PA, McMcormack WM. Risk of acquiring gonorrhea and prevalence of abnormal adnexal findings among women recently exposed to gonorrhea. *JAMA* 1983;**250**:3205–3209.

77. Heinonnen PK, Teisala K, Punnonen R, Miettinen A, Lehtinen M, Paavonen J. Anatomic sites of upper genital tract infection. *Obstet Gynecol* 1985;**66**: 384–390.

78. Cleary RE, Jones RB. Recovery of *Chlamydia trachomatis* from the endometrium in infertile women with serum antichlamydial antibodies. *Fertil Steril* 1985;**44**:233.

79. Spence MR, et al. A comparative evaluation of vaginal, cervical, and peritoneal flora in normal health females. *Sex Transm Dis* 1981;**9**:762.

80. Rank RG, Sanders MM. Ascending genital tract infection as a common consequence of vaginal inoculations with the guinea pig inclusion conjunctivitis agent in normal guinea pigs, in Bowie WR, Caldwell HD, Jones RP, et al. (eds): *Chlamydial Infections. Proceedings of the Seventh International Symposium in Human Chlamydial Infections.* Cambridge, Cambridge Univ. Press, 1990, pp 249–252.

81. Odeblad E. The functional structure of human cervical mucus. *Acta Obstet Gynecol Scand* 1968;**47**(suppl 1):39.

82. Cramer DW, Goldman MB, Schiff I, et al. The relationship of tubal infertility to barrier-method and oral contraceptives use. *JAMA* 1987;**257**:2446–2450.

83. Cates W, Joesoef MR, Goldman MB. Atypical pelvic inflammatory disease: Can we identify clinical predictors? *Am J Obstet Gynecol* 1993;**169**:341–346.

84. Li D-K, Daling JR, Stergachis AS, Chu J, Weiss NS. Prior condom use and the risk of tubal pregnancy. *Am J Public Health* 1990;**80**:964–966.

85. Duncan ME, Tibaux G, Pelzer A, et al. First coitus before menarche and risk of sexually transmitted disease. *Lancet* 1990;**335**:338–340.

86. Rolfs RT, Galaid EI, Zaidi AA. Epidemiology of pelvic inflammatory disease: Trends in hospitalizations and office visits, 1979–1988. *Am J Obstet Gynecol* 1992;**166**:983–990.

87. Forrest KA, Washington AE, Daling JR, Sweet RL. Vaginal douching as a possible risk factor for pelvic inflammatory disease. *J Natl Med Assoc* 1989;**81**:159–165.

88. WHO Scientific Group. The mechanism of action, safety, and efficacy of intrauterine devices. *WHO Tech Rep Ser 753*; 1987.

89. Sweet RL, Blankfort-Doyle M, Robbie MO, Schacter J. The occurrence of chlamydial and gonococcal salpingitis during the menstrual cycle. *JAMA* 1986;**255**:2062–2064.

90. Eschenbach DA, Harnisch JP, Holmes KK. Pathogenesis of acute pelvic inflammatory disease: Role of contraception and other risk factors. *Am J Obstet Gynecol* 1977;**128**:838–850.

91. Masters W, Johnson V. *Human Sexual Response.* Boston, Little Brown, 1966, p 116.

92. Bengtsson LP. Hormonal effects on human myometrial activity. *Vitam Horm* 1973;**31**:257.

93. Filer RB, Wu CH. Coitus during menses: Its effect on endometriosis and pelvic inflammatory disease. *J Reprod Med* 1989;**34**:887–890.

94. Senanayake P, Kramer DG. Contraception and the etiology of pelvic inflammatory disease: New perspectives. *Am J Obstet Gynecol* 1980;**138**:852–860.

95. Svensson L, Weström L, Mardh P. Contraceptives and acute salpingitis. *JAMA* 1984;**251**:2553.

96. Rubin GL, Ory HW, Layde PM. Oral contraceptives and pelvic inflammatory disease. *Am J Obstet Gynecol* 1982;**144**:630.

97. Targum SD, Wright NH. Association of the intrauterine device and pelvic inflammatory disease: A retrospective pilot study. *Am J Epidemiol* 1974;**100**:262–271.

98. Faulkner WL, Ory HW. Intrauterine devices and pelvic inflammatory disease. *JAMA* 1976;**235**:1851–1853.

99. Ryden G, Fahraeus L, Molin L, et al. Do contraceptives influence the incidence of acute pelvic inflammatory disease in women with gonorrhea? *Contraception* 1979;**20**:149–157.

100. Noonan AS, Adams JB. Gonorrhea screening in an urban hospital family planning program. *Am J Public Health* 1974;**64**:700–704.

101. Wølner-Hanssen P. Oral contraceptive use modifies the manifestations of pelvic inflammatory disease. *Br J Obstet Gynecol* 1986;**93**:619–624.

102. Wølner-Hanssen P, Svensson L, Mardh P-H, et al. Laparoscopic findings and contraceptive use in women with signs and symptoms suggestive of acute salpingitis. *Obstet and Gynecol* 1985;**66**:233–238.

103. Oriel JD, Powis PA, Reeve P, et al. Chlamydial infections of the cervix. *Br J Vener Dis* 1974;**50**:11–16.

104. Oriel JD, Johnson AL, Barlow D, et al. Infection of the uterine cervix with *Chlamydia trachomatis. J Infect Dis* 1978;**52**:698–702.

105. Arya OP, Mallison H, Goddard AD. Epidemiological and clinical correlates of chlamydial infection of the cervix. *Br J Vener Dis* 1981;**57**:118–124.

106. Wølner-Hanssen P, Kiviat NB, Holmes KK. Atypical pelvic inflammatory disease: Subacute, chronic, or subclinical upper genital tract infection in women, in Holmes KK, Mardh P-A, Sparling PF, et al. (eds): *Sexually Transmitted Diseases*, 2nd ed. New York, McGraw-Hill, 1990, pp 615–620.

107. Washington AE, Gore S, Schachter J, et al. Oral contraceptives, *Chlamydia trachomatis* infections and pelvic inflammatory diseases. *JAMA* 1985;**253**:2246–2250.

108. Weström L. Incidence, prevalence, and trends of acute pelvic inflammatory disease and its consequences in industrialized countries. *Am J Obstet Gynecol* 1980;**138**:880–892.

109. Buchan H, Villard-Mackintosh L, Vessey M, Yeates D, McPherson K. Epidemiology of pelvic inflammatory disease in parous women with special reference to intrauterine device use. *Br J Obstet Gynaecol* 1990;**97**:780–788.

110. Scholes D, Daling JR, Stergachis AS. Cigarette smoking and risk of pelvic inflammatory disease. *Am J Epidemiol* 1990;**132**:759.

111. Fullilove RE, Fullilove MT, Bowser BP, Gross SA. Risk of sexually transmitted disease among black adolescent crack users in Oakland and San Francisco, Calif. *JAMA* 1990;**263**:851–855.

112. Kronmal RA, Whitney CW, Mumford SD. The intrauterine device and pelvic inflammatory disease: The Woman's Health Study reanalyzed. *J Clin Epidemiol* 1991;**44**:109–122.

113. DATTA panelists. Diagnostic and therapeutic technology assessment. Intrauterine devices. *JAMA* 1989;**261**:2127–2130.

114. Grimes DA. The intrauterine device, pelvic inflammatory disease, and infertility: The confusion between hypothesis and knowledge [comment]. *Fertil Steril* 1992;**58**:670–673.

115. Chi I. What we have learned from recent IUD studies: a researcher's perspective. *Contraception* 1993;**48**:81–108.
116. Weström L, Joesoef R, Reynolds G, Hagdu A, Thompson SE. Pelvic inflammatory disease and fertility. A cohort study of 1,844 women with laparoscopically verified disease and 657 control women with normal laparoscopic results. *Sex Transm Dis* 1992;**19**:185–192.
117. Chow W-H, Daling JR, Weiss NS, et al. Maternal cigarette smoking and tubal pregnancy. *Obstet Gynecol* 1988;**71**:167–170.
118. Phipps WR, Cramer DW, Schiff I, et al. The association between smoking and female infertility as influenced by cause of the infertility. *Fertil Steril* 1987; **48**:377–382.
119. Harlap S, Kost K, Forrest JD. *Preventing Pregnancy, Protecting Health: A New Look at Birth Control Choices in the United States.* New York, The Alan Guttmacher Institute, 1991.
120. Miettinen A, Heinonnen PK, Teisala K, Hakkarainen K, Punnonen R. Serologic evidence for the role of *Chlamydia trachomatis, Neisseria gonorrhoeae,* and *Mycoplasma hominis* in the etiology of tubal factor infertility and ectopic pregnancy. *Sex Transm Dis* 1990;**17**:10–14.
121. Chow JM, Yonekura L, Richwald GA, Greenland S, Sweet RL, Schachter J. The association between *Chlamydia trachomatis* and ectopic pregnancy: A matched-pair, case-control study. *JAMA* 1990;**263**:3164–3167.
122. Chow W-H, Daling JR, Weiss NS, Moore DE, Soderstrom R. Vaginal douching as a potential risk factor for tubal ectopic pregnancy. *Am J Obstet Gynecol* 1985;**153**:727–729.
123. Jones RB, Ardery BR, Hui SL, Cleary RE. Correlation between serum antichlamydial antibodies and tubal factor as a cause of infertility. *Fertil Steril* 1982;**38**:553–558.
124. Moore RE, Spandoni LR, Foy HM, Wang S-P, Daling JR. Recovery of *Chlamydia trachomatis* in infertility due to distal tube disease. *Lancet* 1982;**2**:574–577.
125. Svensson L, Mardh P-A, Ahlgren M, Nordenskjold F. Ectopic pregnancy and antibodies to *Chlamydia trachomatis. Fertil Steril* 1985;**44**:313–317.
126. Aral SO, Cates W. The multiple dimensions of sexual behavior as risk factor for sexually transmitted disease: The sexually experienced are not necessarily sexually active. *Sex Trans Dis* 1989;**12**:173–177.
127. Cates W Jr, Wasserheit JN. Gonorrhea, chlamydia, and pelvic inflammatory disease: A review of the recent literature. *Curr Opin Infect Dis* 1992.
128. Seidman SN, Mosher WD, Aral SO. Predictors of high-risk behavior in unmarried American women: Adolescent environment as risk factor. *J Adolesc Health* 1994;**15**:126–132.
129. Seidman SN, Rieder RO. A review of sexual behavior in the United States. *Am J Psychiatry* 1994;**151**:330–341.
130. Rolfs RT. Personal communication, 1992.
131. Aral SO. Sexual behavior and risk for sexually transmitted infections. *STD Bull* 1991;**10**:3–10.
132. Spence MR, Adler J, McLellan R. Pelvic inflammatory disease in the adolescent. *J Adolesc Health Care* 1990;**11**:304–309.

133. Seidman SN, Aral SO. Sub-population differentials in STD transmission (letter). *Am J Pub Health* 1992;**82**:1297.
134. Wasserheit JN. STD research strategies. *Presented at International STD Research Workship: Priorities for the Agency for International Development in the 1990s.* Centers for Disease Control, Atlanta, Georgia, July 23–25, 1991.
135. McCormack WM. Pelvic inflammatory disease. *N Engl J Med* 1994;**330**: 115–119.

Index

A

Actinomyces israeli, 49, 99
Adnexal masses, and PID, 62
Adolescents and PID, 3
  behavioral risk factors, 119
  biological risk factors, 122
  clinical signs, 125
  complications of, 132–133
  consent for treatment, 125–126
  and contraception method, 119–121
  diagnosis of, 124–127
  differential diagnosis, 128, 131
  epidemiology, 116–119
  and ethnicity, 121–122
  history of patient, taking of, 126–127
  increased risk of PID, 116
  laboratory tests, 130
  long-term sequelae, 133–134
  microbial etiology, 123–124
  pathogenesis, 124
  physical assessment, 129–130
  prevention of, 134–135, 147
  and substance use, 121
  symptoms of PID, 127–129
  treatment of, 131–132
Age
  and PID, 1, 3–4, 193
  and PID sequelae, 27, 162
Amenorrhea, 126
Aminoglycoside, 88, 101, 113, 131
  cautions in pregnancy, 113
Anaerobic/aerobic bacteria, 41–49
  and ectopic pregnancy, 159
  and infertility, 155–156

polymicrobial etiology of PID,
    45–46, 47, 78
  types of, 41–42, 44–46, 78
Antibiotics, 77, 79, 80, 131–132
  antimicrobial activity of regimens, 87
  CDC recommendations, 131
  Chlamydia trachomatis treatment,
    89–90
  combinations used, 84–89
  and cure rates, 85–86
  efficacy of use, 88
  and PID in pregnancy, 112–113
  tubo-ovarian abscess, 100

B

Bacterial vaginosis (BV), 181
Bacteroides fragilis, 99
Barrier contraception
  and adolescents, 120
  effectiveness against STDs, 120
  protection against PID, 11
Blood tests, 63–64
  types of, 63–64

C

Cefotetan, 84, 101
Cefoxitin, 84, 85, 101
Cephalosporin, 88, 113
Cervical discharge, 129–130
Cervical infection, causes of, 1–2
Cervical mucus studies, 64
Chlamydia trachomatis, 1, 3, 4, 5, 6, 8,
    10–11, 12, 13, 14, 36–41
  in adolescents, 116–117

animal studies, 170–171
antibiotic treatment, 89–90
and ectopic pregnancy, 157–158
and endocervicitis, 172–173
and endometritis, 173–176
genital tract changes, 171–172
and infertility, 38–40, 154–155
inflammatory response, 41
and intrauterine device, 13–14
as major causation of PID, 36–40
prior infection and PID, 10–11
and salpingitis, 176–177
spread of, 39–40
tissue damage from, 40–41
Chronic pelvic pain, 159–160
Cigarette smoking
  and infertility, 7
  and PID, 6–7, 123, 149, 190
  and sexually transmitted disease, 6
Ciprofloxicin, 113
Clindamycin, 85, 88, 101, 113, 131
Computed tomography, tubo-ovarian
  abscess, 97–98
Consent, and adolescents, 125–126
Contraception
  adolescent use of, 119–121
  barrier methods, 11
  intrauterine device, 12–14
  oral contraceptives, 11–12
C-reactive protein (CRP), 96
Culdocentesis, 65
Curtis-Fitz-Hugh Syndrome. *See*
  Perihepatitis
Cytomegalovirus, 50

D
Diagnosis of PID, 63–72, 124–125
  blood tests, 63–64
  cervical/vaginal smears, 64–65, 130
  culdocentesis, 65
  differential diagnosis, 70–71
  endometrial biopsy, 68–69
  laparoscopy, 66–68
  microbiological workup, 65
  physical assessment, 129–130
  silent PID, 72
  ultrasonography, 69–70
  urine tests, 63
Douching, and PID, 7–8, 26–27, 123,

149, 162, 189
Doxycycline, 84, 85, 86, 113, 131
Duration of infection, 24–25
Dysmenorrhea, 126

E
Ectopic pregnancy, 156–159
  and adolescents, 133
  and anaerobes, 159
  and chlamydial infections, 157–158
  and concurrent infection, 159
  death rate from, 133
  follow-up studies, 157
  increase in, 133, 156
  and mycoplasma, 158, 159
  and PID, 1, 30
  sites for, 156
Endocervicitis, and *Chlamydia
  trachomatis*, 172–173
Endometrial biopsy, 68–69
Endometritis
  and *Chlamydia trachomatis*, 173–176
  diagnosis of, 69
Erythrocyte sedimentation rate (ESR),
  63–64, 96, 141
Escherichia coli, 31, 44, 99
Ethnicity, and adolescents and PID,
  121–122

F
Fertility
  improvement and PID treatment,
    79–80
  and tubo-ovarian abscess, 103–104
  See also Infertility
Fever, 62, 128–129
Fitz-Hugh-Curtis Syndrome. *See*
  Perihepatitis

G
Gardnerella vaginalis, 31, 44, 47, 122,
  129
Gastrointestinal symptoms, 61, 129
Gentamicin, 85, 101, 113

H
Haemophilus influenzae, 31
Health-care behavior, and PID, 5–6
Herpes simplex virus, 50

History of patient, adolescents,
126–127
HIV and PID, 14, 139–144
clinical course of, 142–143
diagnosis of, 141–142
prevalence of, 140
risk factors, 140
and surgery, 143
treatment of, 143
Hospitalization for PID, 77, 82–84
adolescents, 117, 118, 131
criteria for, 84
decline in, 117, 118
Human immunodeficiency virus (HIV).
See HIV and PID

I

Infertility, 152–156, 190–191
and anaerobes, 156
and chlamydial infections, 154–155
and *Chlamydia trachomatis*,
38–40
and cigarette smoking, 7
and concurrent PID, 152–154
follow-up studies, 154
and intrauterine device, 14
and *Mycoplasma hominis*, 155–
156
and PID, 1, 6, 133–134
See also Fertility
Intrauterine device (IUD)
adolescent use of, 121
Dalkon Shield, 121, 161, 191
disruption of host defense
mechanisms, 48
and infertility, 14
and PID, 12–14, 27, 62, 161
and salpingitis, 48
and tubo-ovarian abscess, 94

L

Laparoscopy, 66–68
and adolescents, 124–125, 131
criticisms of, 68
diagnostic value of, 66, 67–68
and lower abdominal pain, 68
for perihepatitis, 67
and PID in pregnancy, 112
for salpingitis, 66, 125

M

Magnetic resonance imaging (MRI),
tubo-ovarian abscess, 98
Males, and transmission of PID, 5
Menorrhagia, 126
Menstruation
abnormal bleeding, 61, 126
menstrual history of adolescent,
126–127
and PID, 8–9
Metronidazole, 85, 86, 101
Microbial etiology of PID
anaerobic/facultative bacteria, 41–49
Chlamydia trachomatis, 36–41
genital tract mycoplasmas, 49–50
Neisseria gonorrhoeae, 33–36
polymicrobial etiology, 45–46, 47
scope of organisms, 31
spread of organisms, 31–33, 78
and treatment, 30
viruses, 50
Mycoplasmas of genital tract, 49–50,
124
and ectopic pregnancy, 158, 159
and infertility, 155–156
and PID, 49–50
types of organisms, 49

N

Neisseria gonorrhoeae, 1, 3, 4–6, 8, 10,
13, 33–36
in adolescents, 116–118
animal models, 171
genital tract changes, 171–172
in HIV women, 141
inherent properties and infection,
35–36
and intrauterine device, 13–14
and menstrual cycle, 34–35
pathogenic mechanisms, 34–35
prior infection and PID, 10
route of infection, 33–34

O

Ofloxacin, 85, 113
Oral contraceptives
adolescent use of, 120–121
and prevention of PID, 26, 148, 161–
162

and risk of PID, 11–12, 26, 33, 62, 120

P

Pain, 70–71, 127–128
  chronic pelvic pain after PID, 159–160
  diagnosis of, 70–71
  location in PID, 127
  of PID, 60–61
Pelvic inflammatory disease (PID)
  and age, 1, 3–4
  causal factors, 1–2
  chronic pelvic pain after, 159–160
  contraceptive protection against, 11–12
  diagnosis of, 63–72
  duration of infection, 24–25
  and ectopic pregnancy, 156–159
  and health-care behavior, 5–6, 193–194
  and HIV, 14
  and infertility, 152–156
  and menstruation, 8–9
  natural history time line, 21–22
  prevalence of, 1, 30
  prevention of, 76, 134–135, 146–150
  progression of, 183–196
  repetitive infections, factors related to, 9–11, 28, 123
  silent PID, 31
  and socioeconomic status, 2
  symptoms of, 60–63
Pelvic inflammatory disease (PID) risk factors, 23–28
  behavioral risk factors, 24
  Chlamydia trachomatis, 1, 3, 4, 5, 6, 8, 10–11, 12, 13, 14
  cigarette smoking, 6–7
  clinician practices, 28
  douching, 7–8, 26–27
  infectivity rate, 24
  intrauterine device, 12–14, 27
  Neisseria gonorrhoeaa, 1, 3, 4–6, 8, 10, 13
  for PID sequelae, 27–28
  sex partner selection, 23–24
  sexual behavior, 4–5

sociocultural context, 25
Pelvic inflammatory disease (PID) sequelae, 133–134, 152–164
  and age, 162
  animal models, 163
  chronic pelvic pain, 159–160
  and contraception used, 161–162
  and douching behavior, 162
  ectopic pregnancy, 156–159
  future research issues, 163–164
  infertility, 152–156
  and timing of diagnosis/treatment, 162
  and type of organism, 160
Penicillin, 88, 113
Peptostreptococci, 31, 41, 43, 44
Perihepatitis, 132–133
  laparoscopy for, 67
  signs of, 132–133
Polymorphonuclear leukocytes (PMNs), 33, 64, 170–171
Pregnancy and PID
  abortion rate in, 112
  diagnosis of, 110–112
  differential diagnosis, 111
  pathophysiology, 109–110
  reported cases, studies, 108
  treatment, 112–113
Pregnancy test, 63, 130
Prevention of PID, 146–150, 194–195
  and adolescents, 134–135
  awareness/avoidance of risk factors, 148–149
  delaying onset of sexual activity, 147
  factors non amenable to, 147
  and family setting, 150
  goals of, 146, 149
  levels of, 76
  and male partner, 148
  and oral contraceptives, 26, 148
  primary prevention, 134
  regular screening, 147
  secondary prevention, 135
  tertiary prevention, 135
Prevotella species, 31, 41, 44, 47, 99
Progression of PID
  acquisition of lower genital tract infection, 185–187

ascendance to upper genital tract, 188–190
exposure to pathogens, 183–185
female factors, 185
progression to tubal damage, 190–191
Puberty, and risk of PID, 122

R

Recurrent infections, 9–11, 28, 123
Risk factors. *See* Pelvic inflammatory disease (PID) risk factors

S

Salpingitis
animal studies, 170
blood studies, 64
and *Chlamydia trachomatis*, 176–177
and intrauterine device, 48
laparoscopy for, 66, 125
and mycoplasmas of genital tract, 49
proximal stump salpingitis, 63
tubal ligation as protection, 63
Serum IgA antibodies, 64
Serum IgG antibodies, 64
Sex partners, treatment of, 89–90
Sexual behavior
and adolescents, 119
multiple partners, effects of, 4
and PID, 4–5
Sexually transmitted disease (STD)
and cigarette smoking, 6–7
prevention of, 146–150
risk to adolescents, 119
types of organisms, 140
Silent PID, 31, 62–63, 72, 192
diagnosis of, 72
and infertility, 62, 72, 134
signs of, 72
Socioeconomic status, and PID, 2, 191–193
Spermicide, 120, 187
Streptococcus group B, 44
Substance use, and adolescents and PID, 121, 190
Surgery
and HIV women, 143
tubo-ovarian abscess, 101–103

Symptoms of PID, 60–63
adnexal masses, 62
and contraceptive use, 62–63
extragenital symptoms, 61
fever, 128–129
gastrointestinal symptoms, 61, 129
pain, 60–61, 127–128
during physical examination, 62

T

Tetracycline, 88, 113
cautions in pregnancy, 113
Treatment of PID
ambulatory versus hospitalization, 77, 82–84
antibiotics, 77, 79, 80, 84–89
conservative treatment, results of, 79
and culture results, 65
cure rates, 85–86
early, importance of, 81–82
and fertility improvement, 79–80, 81–82
goals of, 76–77, 79
and gonococcal versus nongonococcal infection, 81
sex partners, treatment of, 89–90
successful treatment, signs of, 77
treatment schedules, 83
Tubal factor infertility. *See* Infertility
Tubal ligation, salpingitis protection, 63
Tubo-ovarian abscess, 94–104
in adolescents, 132
antibiotics, 100
differential diagnosis, 96
and fertility, 103–104
imaging methods, 96–98, 130
and intrauterine device, 94
laboratory tests, 96
microbiology, 98–99
pathogenesis, 95
signs of, 96
surgery, 101–103

U

Ultrasonography, 69–70, 130–131
criteria for PID, 69
tubo-ovarian abscess, 96–97, 130

V
Vaginal discharge, 61, 129
Vaginal smears, 64–65
Viruses, in PID, 50

W
White blood cell count, 63, 96

ISBN 0-387-94462-1

EAN

9 780387 944623 >

Pelvic Inflammatory Disease

Springer
*New York
Berlin
Heidelberg
Barcelona
Budapest
Hong Kong
London
Milan
Paris
Santa Clara
Singapore
Tokyo*